Sarcoidosis - New Perspectives

Edited by Seyyed Shamsadin Athari and Entezar Mehrabi Nasab

Published in London, United Kingdom

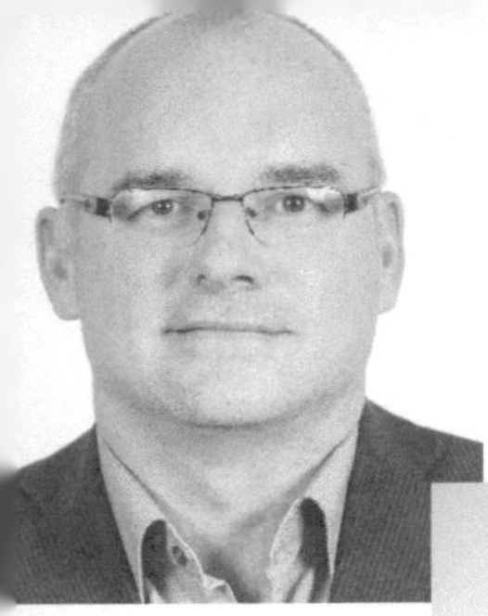
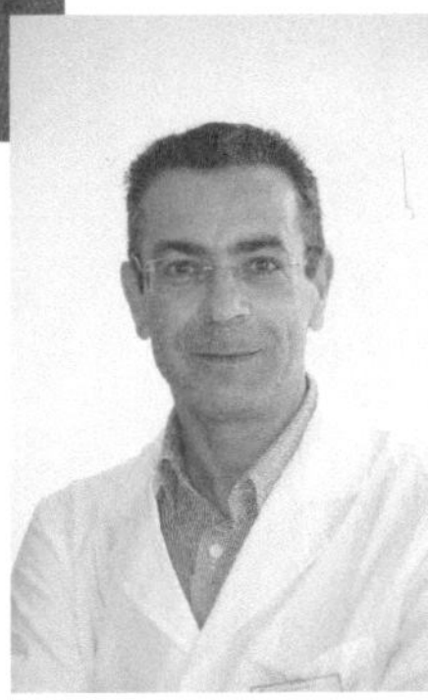
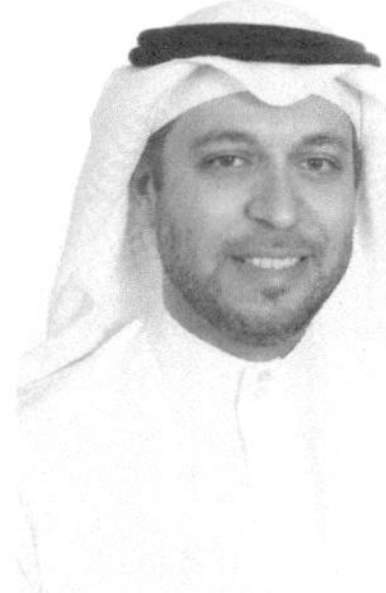
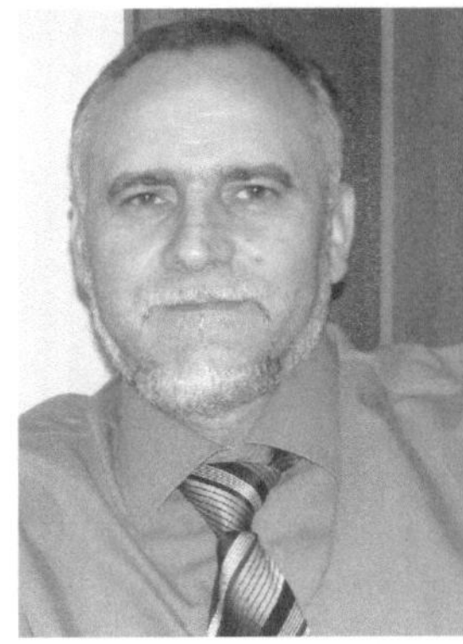
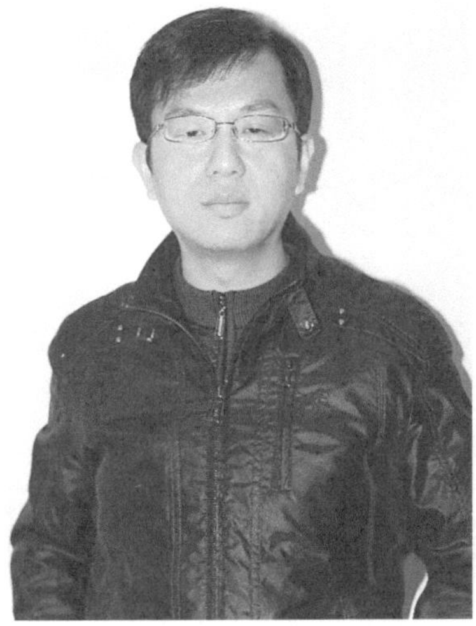
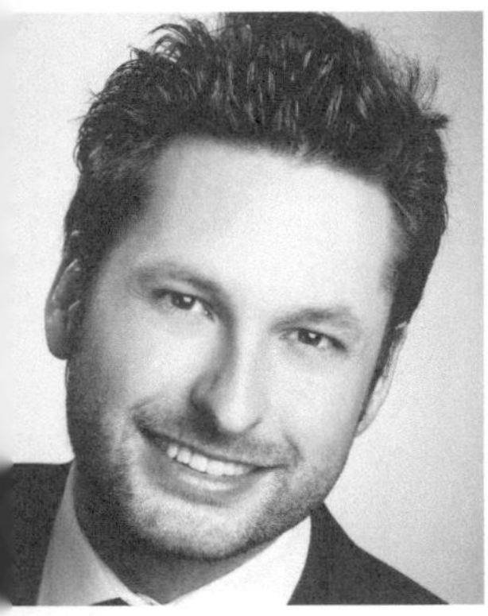
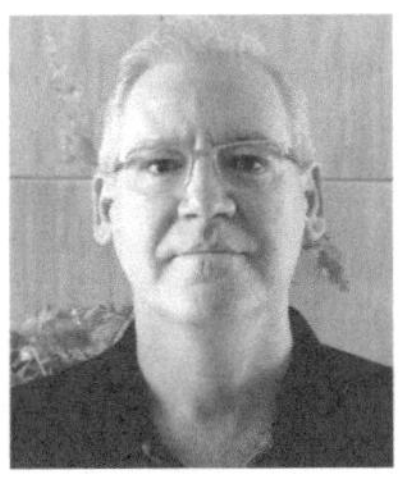

IntechOpen

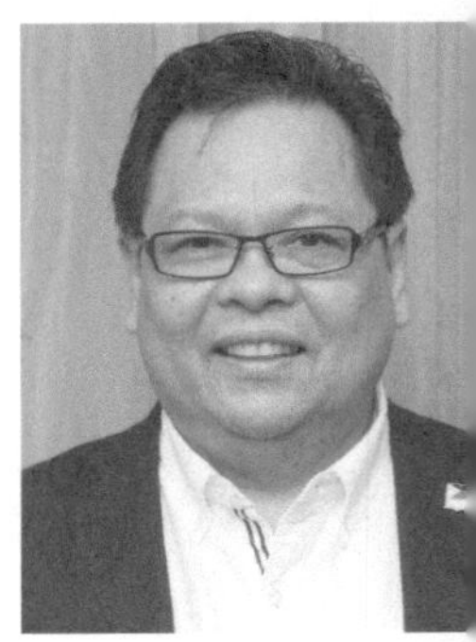
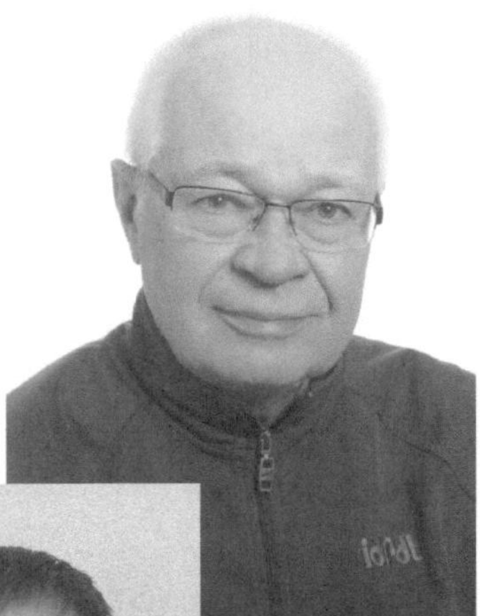
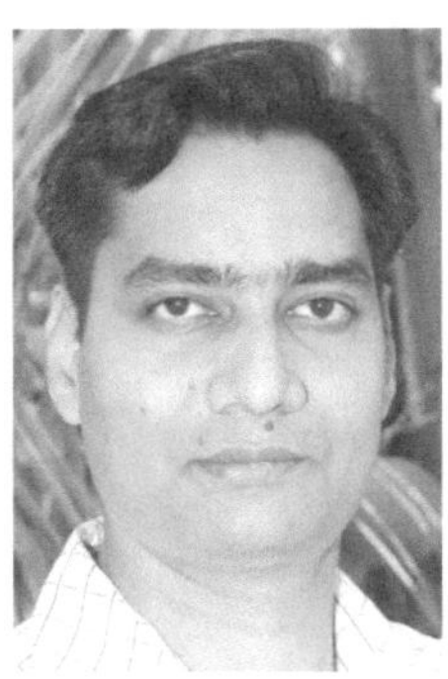
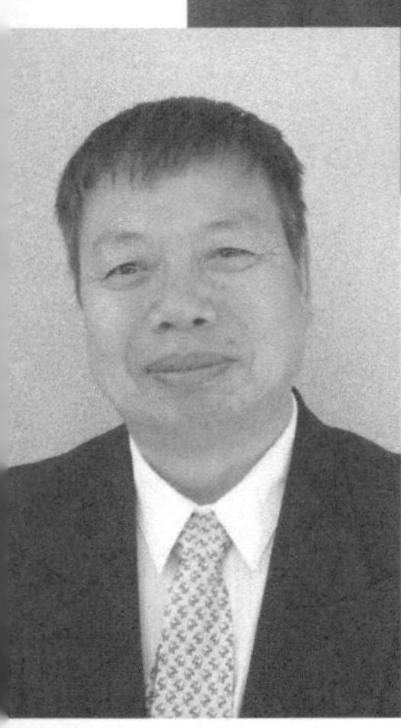
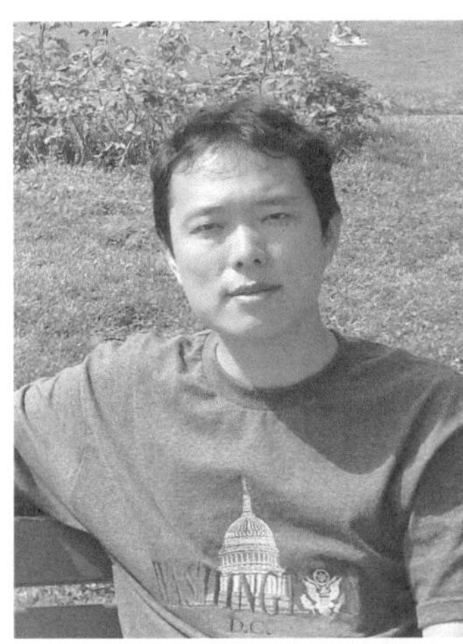
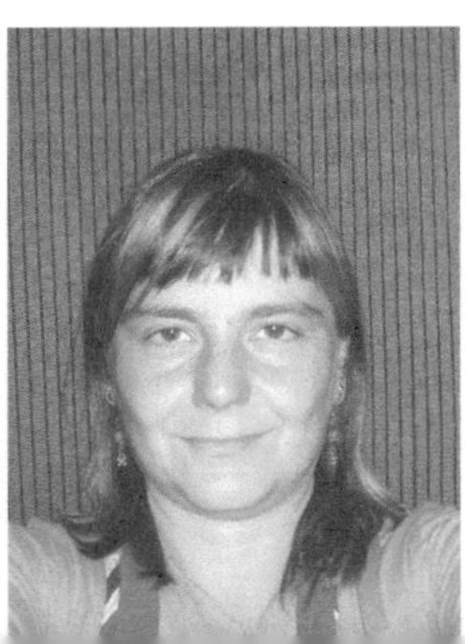

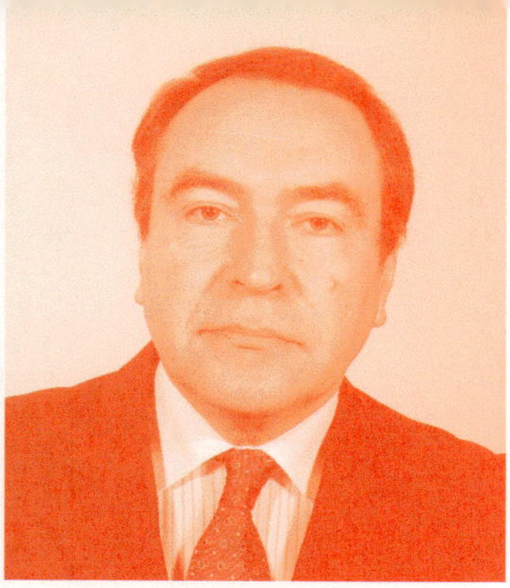

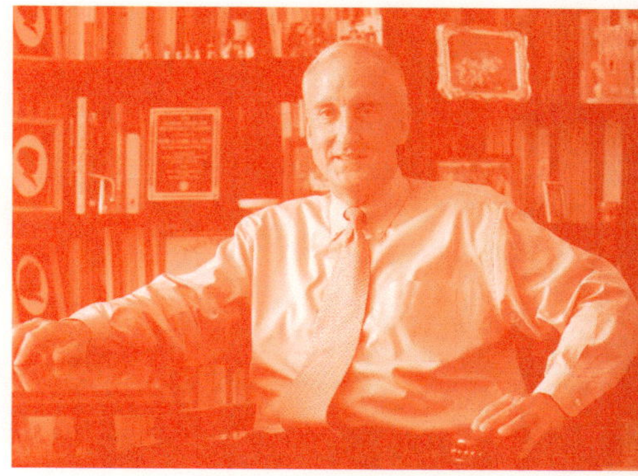

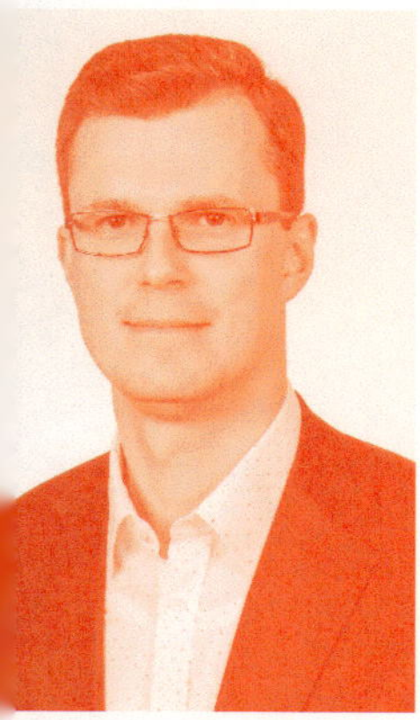

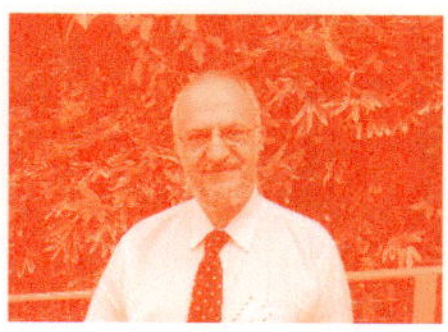

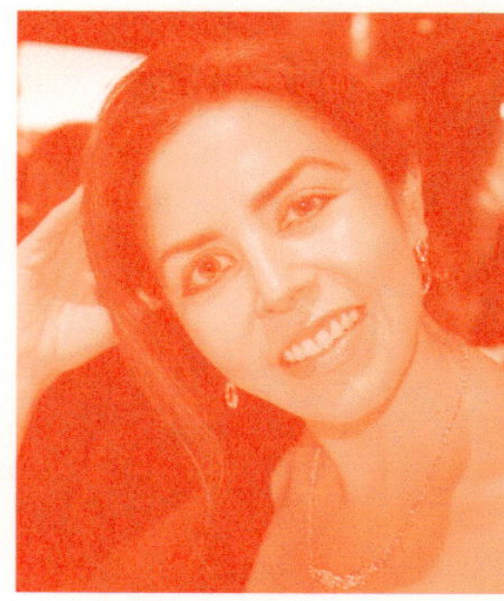

Supporting open minds since 2005

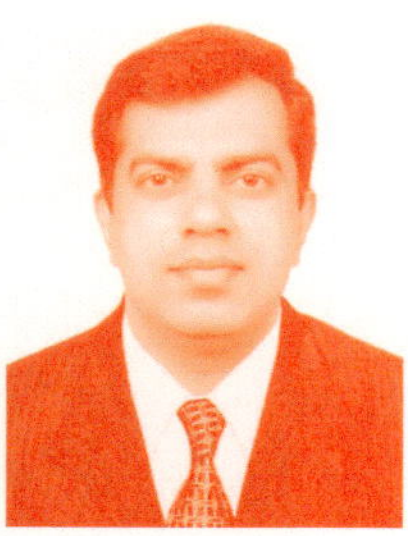

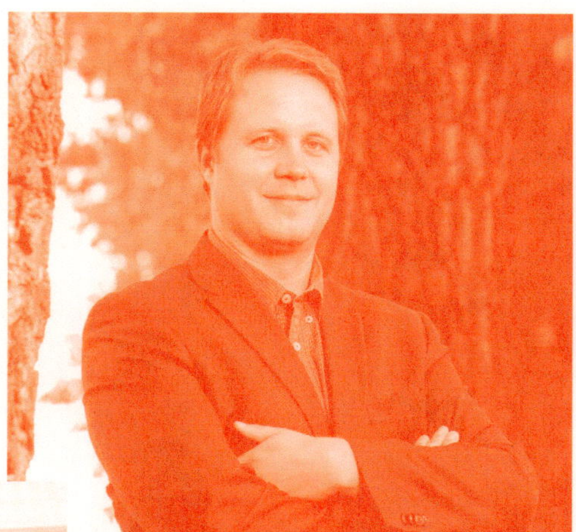

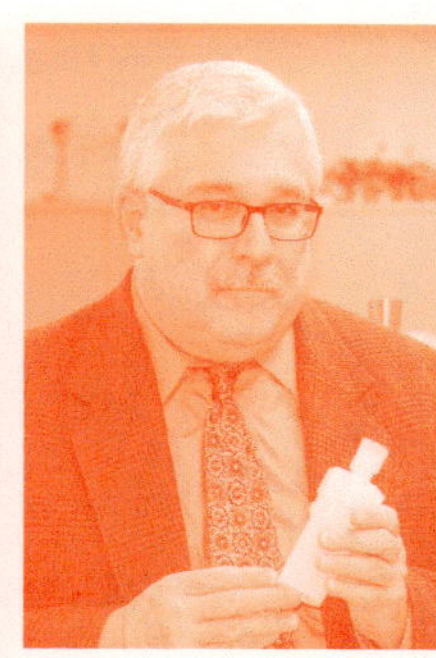

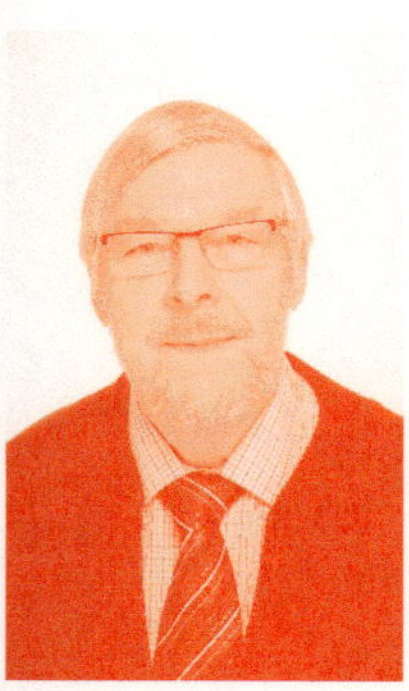

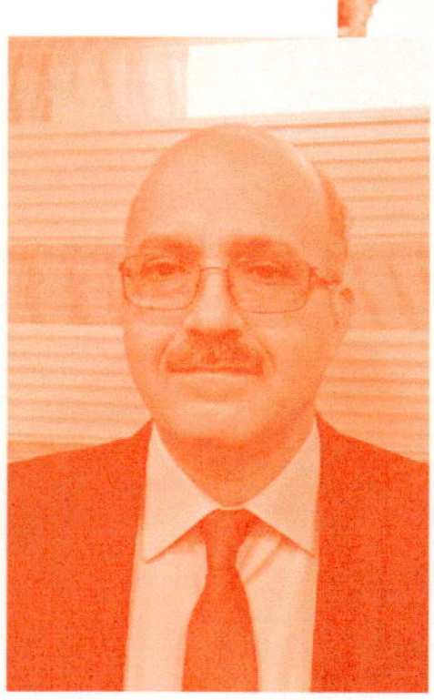

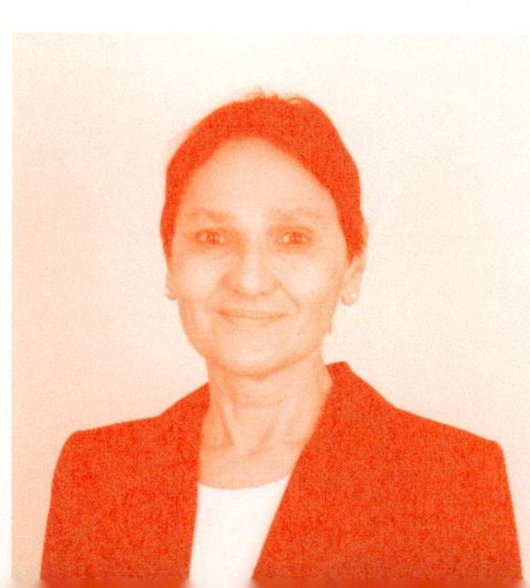

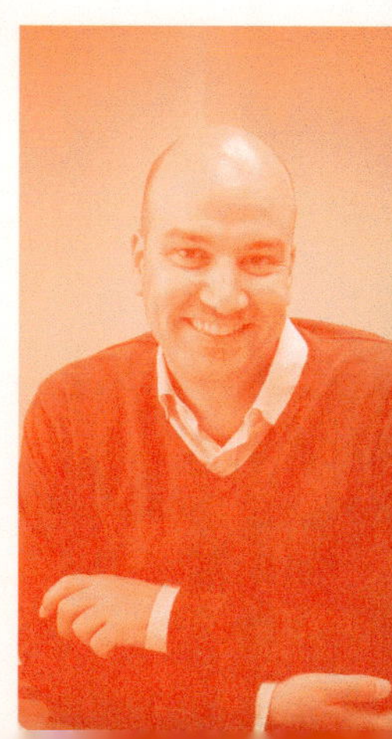

Sarcoidosis - New Perspectives
http://dx.doi.org/10.5772/intechopen.92488
Edited by Seyyed Shamsadin Athari and Entezar Mehrabi Nasab

Contributors
Patricia Lopez Arribas, Álvaro Zapico Goñi, Maria Elena Martínez Gómez, Henco Nel, Eli Gabbay, Aleksandra Speranskaia, Seyyed Shamsadin Athari, Entezar Mehrabi Nasab

First published in London, United Kingdom, 2022 by IntechOpen
IntechOpen is the global imprint of INTECHOPEN LIMITED, registered in England and Wales, registration number: 11086078, 5 Princes Gate Court, London, SW7 2QJ, United Kingdom
Printed in Croatia

British Library Cataloguing-in-Publication Data
A catalogue record for this book is available from the British Library

Additional hard and PDF copies can be obtained from orders@intechopen.com

Sarcoidosis - New Perspectives
Edited by Seyyed Shamsadin Athari and Entezar Mehrabi Nasab
p. cm.
Print ISBN 978-1-83969-917-7
Online ISBN 978-1-83969-918-4
eBook (PDF) ISBN 978-1-83969-919-1

Meet the editors

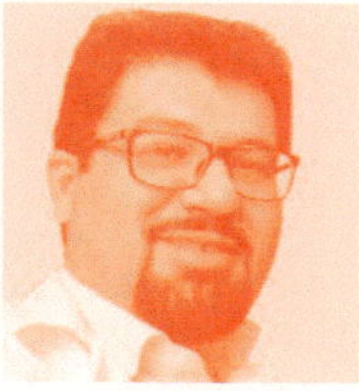

Dr. Seyyed Shamsadin Athari, MPH, Ph.D., is an Assistant Professor of Immunology, Department of Immunology, School of medicine, Zanjan University of Medical Sciences, Iran. He completed postdocs in allergy and asthma toxicology and, asthma management and controlling a network fellowship. He has published more than 30 books and 110 papers in international journals in immunology, allergy, and asthma. He is also on the editorial board of more than seventy journals. He has several scientific inventions to his credit and has recorded gene sequences in a gene bank. Dr. Athari has been invited as a top speaker at more than forty international congresses and symposiums. He is a recipient of several top researcher and young scientist awards.

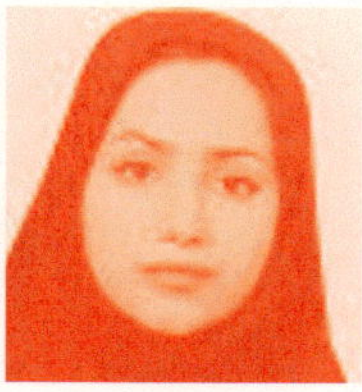

Dr. Entezar Mehrabi Nasab, MD, is a cardiologist specializing in cardiovascular diseases who completed her residency at the Tehran Heart Center, Tehran University of Medical Sciences, Iran. She has published more than twenty scientific articles in international journals. She has been an invited speaker at more than twenty international congresses. Dr. Nasab has received awards from different scientific societies.

Contents

Preface **XI**

Chapter 1 **1**
Introductory Chapter: Sarcoidosis – New Perspectives
by Seyyed Shamsadin Athari and Entezar Mehrabi Nasab

Chapter 2 **5**
Immunopathology of the Sarcoidosis
by Entezar Mehrabi Nasab and Seyyed Shamsadin Athari

Chapter 3 **15**
Mammary Gland Sarcoidosis
by Patricia López Arribas, Maria Elena Martínez Gómez and Alvaro Zapico Goñi

Chapter 4 **23**
Skeletal Sarcoidosis
by Henco Nel and Eli Gabbay

Chapter 5 **35**
Radiation Patterns of Modern Sarcoidosis (Alphabet)
by Aleksandra Speranskaia

Preface

Despite revolutionary advances in medical science, some diseases are still difficult to manage and treat, particularly rare diseases. Thus, much current medical research focuses on identifying molecular mechanisms and cell signaling pathways of disease to develop new treatments. The complexities of pathogenicity and damage of diseases need to be fully understood to design more accurate treatment and control methods.

The immune system is the first line of defense against disease in the human body. Thus, upgrading immune responses is necessary to cure many diseases. In the case of diseases in which infectious agents are involved in pathogenesis, increasing the quality of immune responses sometimes leads to increased resistance to infectious agents and promotes escape routes from the immune system. As such, it is necessary to identify the exact pathways of the immune system to increase the precision of practical responses to diseases such as sarcoidosis.

Sarcoidosis is a rare immune-mediated disease that affects multiple organs in the body. Written by experts in the field, this book presents an overview of the disease from an immunologic perspective. It discusses the cell signaling pathways and molecular mechanisms involved in sarcoidosis as well as pathophysiology, diagnosis, management, and treatment of the disease. The book begins with an introduction to sarcoidosis, including definitions and a description of the disease's immunopathology. Subsequent chapters discuss the disease in more detail as well as highlight recent advances in the field.

The material covered contributes to a better understanding of the immunopathology and molecular pathways of sarcoidosis. This book is a useful resource for researchers and medical professionals both in the lab and in the field.

Dr. Seyyed Shamsadin Athari
Faculty of Medicine,
Department of Immunology,
Zanjan University of Medical Sciences,
Zanjan, Iran

Dr. Entezar Mehrabi Nasab
Department of Cardiology,
School of Medicine,
Tehran Heart Center,
Tehran University of Medical Sciences,
Tehran, Iran

Department of Cardiology,
School of Medicine,
Valiasr Hospital,
Zanjan University of Medical Sciences,
Zanjan, Iran

Chapter 1

Introductory Chapter: Sarcoidosis – New Perspectives

Seyyed Shamsadin Athari and Entezar Mehrabi Nasab

1. Introduction

Sarcoidosis is polygenic, multifactorial, and inflammatory multisystem disease, which preferentially affects the lung and thoracic lymph nodes with the noncaseating epithelioid granulomas formation and is characterized by the presence of noncaseating granulomas. The incidence and prevalence assessment of sarcoidosis is difficult because many patients can be asymptomatic and the disease can also remit spontaneously. In addition to the lungs, the skin, spleen, liver, lymph nodes, heart, and nervous system have all been shown to be affected by sarcoidosis. In 1889, Ernest Besnier described the cutaneous hallmarks of chronic sarcoidosis as lupus pernio. Later, Caesar Boeck used the term sarkoid (sarcoid) for the first time when he observed that the lesions were similar to sarcoma, but benign [1, 2].

2. Sarcoidosis immunopathology

Pathogenesis of sarcoidosis involves both the innate and adaptive immune systems. In patients with sarcoidosis, the activated macrophages and T cells release chemokines and cytokines involved in the formation of the granuloma [such as the tumor necrosis factor-α (TNF-α), interferon-gamma (IFN-γ), interleukin-18 (IL-18), and IL-12]. The clinical appearance of sarcoidosis varies depending on the specific organ involved. It may present with a wide range of clinical functions from asymptomatic to fatal. The sarcoidosis' etiology is still unknown, but many studies have shown that an unknown antigen processed by active macrophages stimulates an immune response that is regulated by T lymphocytes and macrophages. Several studies suggest that not only unknown antigens are responsible for sarcoidosis, but also genetic susceptibility, environmental factors, and in some instances, autoimmunity [2, 3].

Worldwide, the prevalence and incidence of sarcoidosis are not well known. Sarcoidosis affects individuals of all ages irrespective of ethnicity or race, with maximum incidence among people aged 20–39 years, and also, quite more prevalent in nonsmokers, women, and in rural communities. The most common comorbidities encountered in sarcoidosis patients are obesity, coronary heart disease, asthma, hyperlipidemia, diabetes, thyroid disease, osteoporosis, hypertension, chronic renal disease, and chronic obstructive pulmonary disease (COPD). Also, sarcoidosis was often reported in patients with certain autoimmune diseases including Sjogren's syndrome ankylosing spondylitis, autoimmune thyroid disease, and systemic sclerosis. Many studies have hypothesized the role of genetic susceptibility, putative antigens, environmental factors, and autoimmunity in the development of sarcoidosis, but no single cause has been identified to date [2–4]. Although no disease-specific auto-antibodies (Igs) have been observed, it has been presented that the major histocompatibility complex (MHC) class II molecules on antigen-presenting cells (APCs) possess an autoantigen that is recognized by the T cells in sarcoidosis patients. Autoimmunity presents a novel spectrum for immunopathogenesis of sarcoidosis and may help elucidate sarcoid etiology. It was mentioned that sarcoidosis has overlapped with some autoimmune diseases, including autoimmune thyroid disease, rheumatoid arthritis, Sjogren's syndrome, and ankylosing spondylitis; thus, study of the immunopathogenesis of sarcoidosis patients and its correlation with other autoimmune diseases could open new avenues for investigating the underlying causes of this disease [4, 5].

In the most cases in sarcoidosis patients, the growth of these granulomas establishes the primary abnormality. Sarcoid granulomas are ordered, structured masses comprising epithelioid cells, macrophages and their derivatives, giant cells, and T cells. It is presumed that in sarcoidosis, infiltrating T-reg cells fail to reduce the exaggerated inflammatory response, thereby contributing to persistence and integrity of granuloma. Also, T-reg cells release transforming growth factor-β (TGF-β), which may contribute to fibrosis and granuloma. Th17 cells are linked to the sarcoidosis pathogenesis and are recruited to the disease site and involved in the construction of the granuloma. The balance between Th17 and T-reg cells is thought to be disrupted in sarcoidosis and also, is an important factor in sarcoidosis prognosis [2, 4, 6].

Although a wide range of biomarkers has been proposed for screening of sarcoidosis, none is recommended per se in the clinical practice because of the insufficient sensitivity and specificity. Proposed sarcoidosis biomarkers include many cytokines, chemokines, and mediators that are derived from macrophage or and lymphocyte, such as IL-2R, chitotriosidase, neopterin, angiotensin-converting enzyme, and lysozyme, but there is no single reliable biomarker with proven unequivocal prognostic value [1, 3, 4, 6].

Despite extensive research over the past several decades, the sarcoidosis etiology remained unknown. Numerous potential etiological agents have been identified. In recent years, there was an extraordinary increase of data; however, they have very heterogenous characteristics that are used to personalized medicine purpose posing many challenges. The enormous amount of data, applied to the study of sarcoidosis, needs to be dynamically organized and recovered. The integration of the recent deep data will allow to fill the gap between genotype and phenotype, avoiding false-negative and false-positive results. Early diagnosis is important to treat this disease; therefore, there is a fundamental need to develop robust diagnostic tools for the diagnosis and prognosis of sarcoidosis. Recently, new strategies of the sarcoidosis' diagnoses, including FDG-PET scans, HRCT technologies, EBUS, and TBNA, have enhanced the prognosis. More focus should be on the development of noninvasive biomarkers. Corticosteroids play a main role in the treatment of sarcoidosis, but if used for a long time, they can cause many side effects. Second-line and targeted therapies can be promising alternatives for treating sarcoidosis in the near future [5–7]. In this field, precision medicine is the new hope, and it is necessary to be monitored closely for progress toward targeted interventions. For better disease management, multifaceted approaches remain the best practice to ensure competent and effective patient care.

Therefore, in this book, study of new aspect of sarcoidosis was tried, to introduce new way to design advanced methods for prevention, diagnosis, treatment, and control of sarcoidosis.

DOI: http://dx.doi.org/10.5772/intechopen.105554

Author details

Seyyed Shamsadin Athari[1*] and Entezar Mehrabi Nasab[2,3]

1 Faculty of Medicine, Department of Immunology, Zanjan University of Medical Sciences, Zanjan, Iran

2 Tehran Heart Center, Department of Cardiology, School of Medicine, Tehran University of Medical Sciences, Tehran, Iran

3 Department of Cardiology, School of Medicine, Valiasr Hospital, Zanjan University of Medical Sciences, Zanjan, Iran

*Address all correspondence to: ss.athari@gmail.com; ss.athari@zums.ac.ir

References

[1] Sweiss NJ, Salloum R, Gandhi S, Alegre M-L, Sawaqed R, Badaracco M, et al. Significant cd4, cd8, and cd19 lymphopenia in peripheral blood of sarcoidosis patients correlates with severe disease manifestations. PLoS ONE. 2010;**5**(2):e9088

[2] Jain R, Yadav D, Puranik N, Guleria R, Jin J. Sarcoidosis: Causes, diagnosis, clinical features, and treatments. Journal of Clinical Medicine. 2020;**9**:1081

[3] Landi C, Carleo A, Cillis G, Rottoli P. Sarcoidosis: Proteomics and new perspectives for improving personalized medicine. Expert Review of Proteomics. 2018;**15**(10):829-835

[4] Albert M, Adrianto I, Datta I, Iannuzzi MC, Trudeau S, Li J, et al. Association of HLA-DRB1 with sarcoidosis susceptibility and progression in African Americans. American Journal of Respiratory Cell and Molecular Biology. 2015;**53**(2): 206-216

[5] Chen ES, Moller DR. Etiologies of Sarcoidosis. Clinical Reviews in Allergy & Immunology. 2015;**49**(1):6-18

[6] Kiszałkiewicz J, Piotrowski WJ, Brzeziańska-Lasota E. Selected molecular events in the pathogenesis of sarcoidosis – recent advances. Pneumonologia i alergologia polska. 2015;**83**(6):462-475

[7] Wang V, Jiang F, Kallepalli A, Basen T, Yusin J, Krishnaswamy G. Sarcoidosis. Annals of Allergy, Asthma and Immunology. 2018;**121**(6):662-667

Chapter 2

Immunopathology of the Sarcoidosis

Entezar Mehrabi Nasab and Seyyed Shamsadin Athari

Abstract

Sarcoidosis as a multisystemic inflammatory granulomatous disorder is characterized by local immune hyperactivation, inflammation, and granuloma formation. Many organs may be involved by sarcoidosis. The pathogenesis of sarcoidosis may be autoimmune response to an antigenic exposure. The lung is affected in the vast majority of patients, and common symptoms in lung sarcoidosis are nonproductive cough and dyspnea. The death cause is typically severe pulmonary complications, involvement of myocardia, and central nervous system. Sarcoid granuloma is comprised of epithelioid, mononuclear, and CD4+ T cells with a few CD8+ T cells. It was confirmed that there is association between HLA Class I and II genes as risk factors with sarcoidosis. Some alleles have protective effect against immunopathology of sarcoidosis, and some others are risk factor. The immune mechanisms of sarcoidosis are not completely understood. The inflammasome signal transductions pathway plays a critical role in sarcoidosis pathogenesis. Sarcoidosis treatment could potentially benefit from simultaneous modulation and fine-tuning of M2/Th2 and M1/Th1 pathways rather than targeting one pathway or the other. Future experimental investigations and clinical studies into sarcoidosis and all types of sarcoid reaction may increase our understanding.

Keywords: immune response, immune regulation, immune modulation, immunosurveillance

1. Introduction

Sarcoidosis as a multisystemic inflammatory granulomatous disorder is characterized by the mononuclear phagocyte's accumulation, local immune hyperactivation, and non-necrotizing epithelial cell granulomas formation. There is a complex interaction between tissue cells and the adaptive immune systems, notably T lymphocyte, dendritic cells (DCs), cytokines, and immunopathological process. Many organs including lungs and upper respiratory tract, skin, liver, heart, spleen, central nervous system, eyes, mediastinal and peripheral lymph nodes, parotid glands, bones, and joints may be involved by sarcoidosis [1–3].

Noncaseating granuloma is the pathological hallmark of sarcoidosis that is most often associated with lymph node and pulmonary involvement. The granuloma is an immunological response to an unidentified antigenic trigger. Also, recent advances in the genetics of sarcoidosis report considerable variation by population in the genes as well. The pathogenesis of sarcoidosis may be autoimmune response to an antigenic exposure. The T cells role in the antigen's recognition and in the amplification of inflammatory responses was well established and, dendritic cells have a prominent role in the immunopathological processes. For example, in cutaneous lesions of sarcoidosis, histological findings of the sarcoid lesions show that the granulomas center is typically surrounded by T helper (CD4+ lymphocytes), rare T cytotoxic (CD8+ lymphocytes), and mature macrophages. Also, two populations of dendritic cells occur in normal skin: dermal dendritic cells and epidermal Langerhans cells (LCs). LCs are involved in the epidermal microenvironment monitoring by taking up and processing antigen and dermal dendritic cells that are mature antigen-presenting cells (APCs). In primary cutaneous sarcoidosis, increased number of epidermal LCs was reported [2–6].

Thus, the sarcoidosis etiology is complex and likely a heterogeneous group of disorders with a final pathway to inflammable granulomatous with a polygenic inheritance for susceptible individuals [2, 4, 5]. The genetic predisposition may be determined by the effects of several genes that are associated with human leukocyte antigens and various cytokines. A number of immunoglobulin receptor genes have implication in the immune responses regulation and the sarcoidosis pathogenesis.

2. Immunopathology

Sarcoidosis is a rare inflammatory disorder and during the recent decades, the disease became more prevalent, likely due to improvement in imaging modalities. Hence, early recognition of sarcoidosis is imperative to prevent detrimental consequences. On the basis of secreted cytokine, Th cells are divided into two subsets: Th1 and Th2 cells. Th1 cell's cytokines (TNF-α, IL-2, INF-γ, and IL-12) mediate cell-mediated immunity, while Th2 cell's cytokines (IL-4, IL-5, and IL-13) are associated with function for antibody of the B cells. TNF-α plays an important role in cell-mediated immune responses and the Th1 responses development and participates in the induction and maintenance of granulomas. Therefore, inhibition of TNF-α is an effective treatment in sarcoidosis [7, 8].

In sarcoidosis, elevated Th1 cytokines (IL-2, IFN-γ, TNF-α, and IL-12), monocytes/macrophages cytokines (IL-15 and T cell stimulatory cytokine), IL-18, an IFN-γ-enhancing factor contribute to Th1 responses. T cells migrate to the inflammation site, in response to chemoattractant molecules [including CC chemokine ligand (CCL2), monocyte chemoattractant protein (MCP)-1, regulated upon activation, normal T cell expressed and secreted (RANTES) or CCL5, IL-16, macrophage inflammatory protein (MIP)-1α (CCL3), INF-γ-inducible protein (IP)-10 (CX chemokine ligand (CXCL)10), MIP-1β (CCL4), and MIP-3β (CCL19)]. Also, lung-accumulated T cells express Th1-associated chemokine receptors (such as CXCR3 and CCR5) and reduce Th2-associated CCR4 and CXCR4 [9–12].

Sarcoidosis affects virtually any organ. However, the lung is affected in the vast majority of patients, and common symptoms in lung sarcoidosis are nonproductive cough and dyspnea. The death cause is typically severe pulmonary complications, involvement of myocardia, and central nervous system. On the other hand, acute form of Löfgren's syndrome in patients has a good prognosis, especially in HLA-DRB1*03-positive patients. In sarcoidosis, the bronchoalveolar lavage fluid (BALF) shows alveolitis symptoms, increased T CD4+, elevated the CD4/CD8 Ratio, and increased numbers of neutrophils or mast cells. Furthermore, epithelioid cells of the sarcoidosis's granuloma can produce angiotensin-converting enzyme (ACE) that reflect the granuloma burden [2, 4, 13, 14].

T-regulatory (Treg) cells with expression of CD4, CD25 bright, and forkhead boxp3 (FOXP3), are capable of suppressing cytokine production and proliferation of activated T cells. Moreover, Treg cell in sarcoidosis is seemed to be dysfunctional because it inhibits proliferation but not TNF-α and IFN-γ production. The natural killer (NK)T cell have a capacity to produce large quantities of both IFN-γ (Th1) and IL-4 (Th2) cytokines. They recognize glycolipid antigens presented by CD1d molecules, regulate the immune response, and prevent the Th1-mediated autoimmune diseases progression, and the reduced levels of NKT cells in sarcoidosis were reported [15–18].

Sarcoid granuloma is comprised of epithelioid, mononuclear, and CD4+ T cells with a few CD8+ T cells. In sarcoidosis, the B7:CD28/CTLA-4 costimulatory pathway is essential for T cell activation. Activated T cells and macrophages within the granuloma release key inflammatory cytokines. The antigen-presenting cells (APCs) including dendritic cells (DCs) and macrophages within the granuloma are distinguished by the increased presence of anti-follicular dendritic cells 1 RFD1 and RFD7 cell surface markers (RFD1+/D7+ antigen-presenting cells (APCs)) in active sarcoidosis. APCs express peroxisome proliferator-activated receptor (PPAR)g, as a transcription factor, induce macrophage IL-10 production, and inhibit myeloid DC development and function. Moreover, in sarcoidosis, antigen-driven inflammation causes maturation, activation, and migration of DC to the draining lymph nodes driving T cell expansion. Also, activated DCs release the Th1-polarizing inflammatory mediators TNF-α, IL-12, and IL-18. Furthermore, the number of Th17 cells is elevated in lung and bronchoalveolar cells of sarcoidosis patients that suggests that Th17 responses contribute to granulomatous inflammation. In addition, the enhanced expression of a plethora of cytokines including TNF-α, IL-1b, IL-10, IL-12, IL-15, IL-18, and TGF-β has been reported in sarcoidosis [8, 10, 19–24].

Toll-like receptors (TLRs) are responsible for the molecular recognition of pathogens and can initiate the inflammatory immune responses. In general, pathogen-activated molecular patterns (PAMPSs) activation results in the activation of complex signal transduction pathways including that of the inflammasome that are involved in the pathogenesis of sarcoidosis. The NLRP3 inflammasome downstream of TLR activation results in the inflammasome-regulated mediators' expression, IL-1β, IL-18, and IL-33, following caspase 1 cleavage of mediator pro-forms [25–29]. In contrast to apparent depressed cellular immunity, in active sarcoidosis, the humoral immunity is not only intact but also hyperactive. Patients with sarcoidosis have polyclonal elevation of serum immunoglobulins and also increased levels of free light chains (both kappa and lambda). The hyperactivity of the humoral immunity is not limited to peripheral blood but is present in areas of active disease. The patients with pulmonary sarcoidosis have revealed increased numbers of B cells and increased levels of IgG in bronchoalveolar lavage fluid (BALF). The active sarcoidosis is associated with polyclonal hypergammaglobulinemia, which is due to stimulation of B cells, by increased numbers of activated T helper at the sites of active granuloma formation. On the other hand, these immunoglobulins participate in the immune complexes formation with an antigen, which may be self or foreign. Indeed soluble immune complexes are found in both the blood and BALF of patients with active sarcoidosis. It is feasible that these immune complexes precipitate and participate actively in granuloma formation. But, the role of polyclonal hypergammaglobulinemia in the sarcoidosis pathogenesis is unclear [9, 11, 17, 20, 23, 26].

Sarcoidosis has no specific biomarker. Some markers are for sarcoidosis such as angiotensin-converting enzyme (ACE) and lysozyme enzymes produced by macrophages that display low sensitivity and/or specificity in granuloma. During development of granuloma, a number of biomarkers are released by immune cells. CD4+ T cells differentiate into specific subtypes such as Th1, Th2, T follicular helper (Tfh), Th17, Th17.1, and Treg. The Th1, 17, and Th17.1 produce inflammatory markers (i.e. IFN-γ, IL-17A, and IFN-γ/IL-17A, respectively). Through IL-2 production, CD8+ T cells differentiate into cytotoxic T cells and produce inflammatory biomarkers (i.e. perforin and granzyme), while the Th17 attracts neutrophils via CXCL8 and IL-17A, further contributing to inflammatory marker production. The Th2 and Th17 secrete IL-4, IL-13, and TGF-β1, which are biomarkers of fibrosis. The Treg and NKT cells also modulate the CD4+ T cell immune response. M1 macrophages release inflammatory biomarkers [i.e. IL-12, chitotriosidase (CTO), serum amyloid A (SAA), CXCL9, CXCL10, and CXCL11], while M2 macrophages produce fibrosis biomarkers (i.e. CCL18) and TGF-β1) [30–36].

3. Pathogenesis and immunogenesis

Genome-wide association studies (GWASs) confirmed that there is association for HLA Class I and II genes including HLA-B7, HLA-B8, DRB1*03, DRB1*11, DRB1*12, DRB1*14, and DRB1*15 as risk factors in sarcoidosis, and in contrast, HLA-DRB1*01 and DRB1*04 have protective effects against immunopathology of sarcoidosis. Also, two non-HLA associations were determined. The butyrophilin-like 2 (BTNL2) gene as a risk factor is a negative costimulatory molecule, whose lack of function could result in amplified T cell activation. The annexin A11 (ANXA11) as a protective gene has effects on autoantibody production [22, 27, 37–39].

In sarcoidosis, the exact pathogenesis of granuloma formation remains unknown. The cell-mediated delayed-type hypersensitivity immune reaction (type IV hypersensitivity) leads to granuloma formation in the context of immune dysfunction. After presentation of the phagocytized antigen by macrophages, the effector helper T cells CD4+ secrete IL-2 and IFN-γ and induce Th1 immune responses. The collection of inflammatory cells results in the formation of a granuloma by highly differentiated epithelioid cells and giant cells (mononuclear phagocytes) and lymphocytes. However, there is a lack of evidence as to whether some infectious and noninfectious can be identified as the cause of granuloma, despite a variety of proposed causes. Thus, while the involvement of a type IV (Th1-type) hypersensitivity response is being established, the genetic predisposition concept to sarcoidosis susceptibility and the causative antigen nature had not been well defined [14, 18, 25, 33, 38].

The immune mechanisms of sarcoidosis are not completely understood. The inflammasome signal transductions pathway plays a critical role in sarcoidosis pathogenesis. JAK-STAT signaling is strongly implicated in pathogenesis of the sarcoidosis with Signal Transducer and Activator of Transcription 3 (STAT3) and STAT1/STAT4 playing main roles in Th1 and Th17 cell differentiation, respectively. Also, altered mammalian target of rapamycin (mTOR) signaling negatively affects differentiation of Th17 and of Th17-associated inflammatory biomarkers production. Through the expression of inducible costimulator (ICOS) and CD40 ligand (CD40L), the Tfh cells helps B cells differentiation to plasma cells which secrete immunoglobulins to sarcoid antigens [11, 17, 22, 34, 40–42].

Corticosteroids are the first-line therapeutic approach due to potent anti-inflammatory and immune-suppressing actions, which inhibit TNF-α, INF-γ, and related (e.g. NF-κB) signaling pathways. Moreover, immune checkpoint inhibitors suppress immune responses. Programmed cell death protein 1 (PD-1) and its receptor/ligand (PD-L1) as potent immune checkpoint inhibitors are the reversal of immune exhaustion by restoring T cell cytokine responses and proliferation capacity. Likewise, cytotoxic T lymphocyte antigen 4 (CTLA-4) is expressed on activated T cells and inhibits T cell proliferation and activation by blocking B7 with CD28 costimulation. Blocked CTLA-4 increases Th17 while impairing Tregs functions that have important implications for pathogenesis of the sarcoidosis. CTLA-4 expression, therefore, might be a potential therapy in sarcoidosis [5, 9, 14, 26, 37, 43].

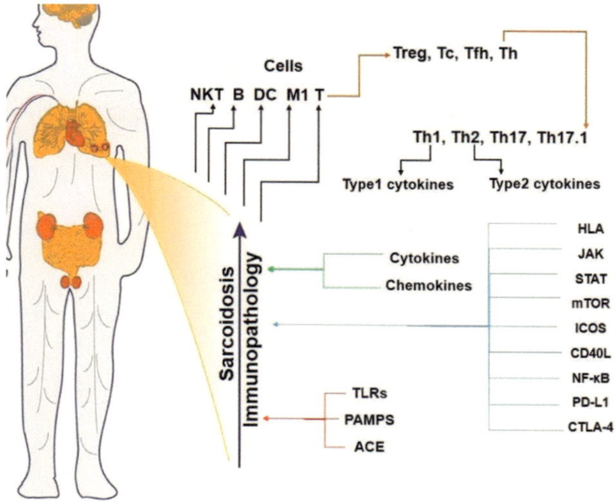

Figure 1.
Immune biomarkers related to immunopathology of sarcoidosis.

The most useful approach to simultaneously diagnose, treat, and predict prognosis in sarcoidosis may be to measure immune system biomarkers in blood or BAL fluid panel. However, in diagnosing sarcoidosis, a comprehensive history and physical exam remains indispensable. Once sarcoidosis-specific biomarkers are determined relative to other conditions, to look for a high percentage of Th1 and Th17 CD4+ cells expressing PD-1, intermediates frequency Th17/Th17.1, and high levels of Treg with increased CD95/CTLA-4 expression in sarcoidosis. Simultaneously increased BAL fluid level of TGF-β1 and CCL18 secreting CCR6+ CD4+ T cells will raise clinical suspicion of fibrosing sarcoidosis. In some patients, anti-inflammatory treatments targeting Th1/M1 immune responses may be benefit, whereas others block regulatory/pro-fibrotic Th2/M2 polarization may be benefit (**Figure 1**). Therefore, sarcoidosis treatment could potentially benefit from simultaneous modulation and fine-tuning of M2/Th2 and M1/Th1 pathways rather than targeting one pathway or the other [17, 23, 30, 44, 45].

4. Conclusion remarkable

During the last decade, there is a pathophysiological rationale for the use of treatments, alone or in combination with other agents to treat sarcoidosis. There appears to be lack of data from prospective studies or clinical trials to prove their efficacy in reversing conduction abnormality, immunopathogenesis, or improving mortality. Currently, there are large knowledge gaps in the field of sarcoidosis and immunotherapeutic agents as new concepts of disease treatment and study of pathogenesis are necessary. A review of the immune aspects of sarcoidosis leaves no doubt that this is a disease promoted by local aberrations in immunological reactivity. Although the initiating factors are not clear, it is now accepted that the development of sarcoidosis is the result of an overstimulated local cellular immune response. Recent results are presented a central role of the immune cells in controlling the course of this disease, interstitial inflammation, and subsequent progression of fibrosis. More researches are necessary to better characterize its immunopathology. In this light, future experimental investigations and clinical studies into sarcoidosis and all types of sarcoid reaction may increase our understanding and, we hope, improve our management of immunity-related disorders.

Author details

Entezar Mehrabi Nasab[1] and Seyyed Shamsadin Athari[2]*

1 Department of Cardiology, School of Medicine, Tehran Heart Center, Tehran University of Medical Sciences, Tehran, Iran

2 Department of Immunology, School of Medicine, Zanjan University of Medical Sciences, Zanjan, Iran

*Address all correspondence to: ss.athari@gmail.com

References

[1] Bordignon M, Rottoli P, Agostini C, Alaibac M. Adaptive immune responses in primary cutaneous sarcoidosis. Clinical and Developmental Immunology. 2011: Article ID 235142

[2] Iannuzzi MC, Rybicki BA, Teirstein AS. Sarcoidosis. New England Journal of Medicine. 2007;**357**(21):2153-2108

[3] Miyara M, Amoura Z, Parizot C, et al. The immune paradox of sarcoidosis and regulatory T cells. Journal of Experimental Medicine. 2006;**203**(2):359-370

[4] Baughman RP, Lower EE, Du Bois RM. Sarcoidosis. Lancet. 2003;**361**(9363):1111-1118

[5] Zissel G, Prasse A, Müller-Quernheim J. Immunologic response of sarcoidosis. Seminars in Respiratory and Critical Care Medicine. 2010;**31**(4):390-403

[6] Noor A, Knox KS. Immuno-pathogenesis of sarcoidosis. Clinics in Dermatology. 2007;**25**(3): 250-258

[7] De Jager M, Blokx W, Warris A, et al. Immunohistochemical features of cutaneous granulomas in primary immunodeficiency disorders: A comparison with cutaneous sarcoidosis. Journal of Cutaneous Pathology. 2008;**35**(5):467-472

[8] Ota M, Amakawa R, Uehira K, et al. Involvement of dendritic cells in sarcoidosis. Thorax. 2004;**59**(5): 408-413

[9] Kataria YP, Holter JF. Immunology of sarcoidosis. Clinics in Chest Medicine. 1997;**18**(4):719-739

[10] Grunewald J. Clinical aspects and immune reactions in sarcoidosis. The Clinical Respiratory Journal. 2007;**1**: 64-73

[11] Mempel M, Flageul B, Suarez F, Ronet C, Dubertret L, Kourilsky P, et al. Comparison of the T cell patterns in leprous and cutaneous sarcoid granulomas. Presence of Valpha 24-invariant natural killer T cells in T-cell-reactive leprosy together with a highly biased T cell receptor Valpha repertoire. The American Journal of Pathology. 2000;**157**:509-523

[12] Ho LP, Urban BC, Thickett DR, Davies RJ, McMichael AJ. Deficiency of a subset of T-cells with immunoregulatory properties in sarcoidosis. Lancet. 2005;**365**: 1062-1072

[13] Kobayashi S, Kaneko Y, Seino K, et al. Impaired IFN-gamma production of Valpha 24 NKT cells in non-remitting sarcoidosis. International Immunology. 2004;**16**:215-222

[14] du Bois RM, Goh N, McGrath D, Cullinan P. Is there a role for microorganisms in the pathogenesis of sarcoidosis? Journal of Internal Medicine. 2003;**253**:4-17

[15] Drake WP, Newman LS. Mycobacterial antigens may be important in sarcoidosis pathogenesis. Current Opinion in Pulmonary Medicine. 2006;**12**:359-363

[16] Mortaz E, Masjedi MR, Tabarsi P, Pourabdollah M, Adcock IM. Immunopathology of Sarcoidosis. Iranian Journal of Allergy, Asthma, and Immunology. 2014;**13**(5):300-306

[17] Agostini C, Trentin L, Facco M, Sancetta R, Cerutti A, Tassinari C, et al. Role of IL-15, IL-2, and their receptors in the development of T cell alveolitis in pulmonary sarcoidosis. Journal of Immunology. 1996;**157**(2):910-918

[18] Moller DR, Forman JD, Liu MC, Noble PW, Greenlee BM, Vyas P, et al. Enhanced expression of IL-12 associated with TH1 cytokine profiles in active pulmonary sarcoidosis. Journal of Immunology. 1996;**156**(12):4952-4960

[19] Newman LS. Aetiologies of sarcoidosis. European Respiratory Monograph. 2005;**32**:23-48

[20] Walker C, Bauer W, Braun RK, Menz G, Braun P, Schwarz F, et al. Activated T cells and cytokines in bronchoalveolar lavages from patients with various lung diseases associated with eosinophilia. American Journal of Respiratory and Critical Care Medicine. 1994;**150**(4):1038-1048

[21] Hauber HP, Gholami D, Meyer A, Pforte A. Increased interleukin-13 expression in patients with sarcoidosis. Thorax. 2003;**58**(6):519-524

[22] Romics L Jr, Dolganiuc A, Velayudham A, Kodys K, Mandrekar P, Golenbock D, et al. Toll-like receptor 2 mediates inflammatory cytokine induction but not sensitization for liver injury by Propioni- bacterium acnes. Journal of Leukocyte Biology. 2005;**78**(6):1255-1264

[23] Yim JJ, Lee HW, Lee HS, Kim YW, Han SK, Shim YS, et al. The association between microsatellite polymorphisms in intron II of the human Toll-like receptor 2 gene and tuberculosis among Koreans. Genes and Immunity. 2006;**7**(2):150-155

[24] Liu H, Komai-Koma M, Xu D, Liew FY. Toll-like receptor 2 signaling modulates the functions of CD4+ CD25+ regulatory T cells. Proceedings of the National Academy of Sciences of the United States of America. 2006;**103**(18):7048-7053

[25] Zhou E-R, Arce S. Key players and biomarkers of the adaptive immune system in the pathogenesis of sarcoidosis. International Journal of Molecular Sciences. 2020;**21**:7398

[26] Heron M, Claessen AM, Grutters JC, van den Bosch JM. T-cell activation profiles in different granulomatous interstitial lung diseases-A Role for CD8+CD28(Null) cells? Clinical and Experimental Immunology. 2010;**160**:256-265

[27] Kamphuis LS, van Zelm MC, Lam KH, Rimmelzwaan GF, Baarsma GS, Dik WA, et al. Perigranuloma localization and abnormal maturation of B cells. American Journal of Respiratory and Critical Care Medicine. 2013;**187**: 406-416

[28] Kudryavtsev I, Serebriakova M, Starshinova A, Zinchenko Y, Basantsova N, Malkova A, et al. Imbalance in B cell and T follicular helper cell subsets in pulmonary sarcoidosis. Scientific Reports. 2020;**10**:1-10

[29] León B, Ballesteros-Tato A, Misra RS, Wojciechowski W, Lund FE. Unraveling eector functions of B cells during infection: The hidden world beyond antibody production. Infectious Disorders Drug Targets. 2012;**12**:213-221

[30] Morita R, Schmitt N, Bentebibel SE, Ranganathan R, Bourdery L, Zurawski G, et al. Human blood CXCR5(+) CD4(+) T cells are counterparts of T follicular cells and contain specific subsets that dierentially support antibody secretion. Immunity. 2011;**34**:108-121

[31] Saussine A, Tazi A, Feuillet S, Rybojad M, Juillard C, Bergeron A, et al. Active chronic sarcoidosis is characterized by increased transitional blood B cells, increased IL-10-producing regulatory B cells and high BAFF levels. PLoS One. 2012;**7**:e43588

[32] Ando M, Goto A, Takeno Y, Yamasue M, Komiya K, Umeki K, et al.

Significant elevation of the levels of B-cell activating factor (BAFF) in patients with sarcoidosis. Clinical Rheumatology. 2018;**37**:2833-2838

[33] Le V, Crouser ED. Potential immunotherapies for sarcoidosis. Expert Opinion on Biological Therapy. 2018;**18**(4):399-407

[34] Wenzel S, Ford L, Pearlman D, et al. Dupilumab in persistent asthma with elevated eosinophil levels. The New England Journal of Medicine. 2013;**368**:2455-2466

[35] Eishi Y, Suga M, Ishige I, et al. Quantitative analysis of mycobacterial and propionibacterial DNA in lymph nodes of japanese and european patients with sarcoidosis. Journal of Clinical Microbiology. 2002;**40**:198-204

[36] Song Z, Marzilli L, Greenlee BM, et al. Mycobacterial catalase-peroxidase is a tissue antigen and target of the adaptive immune response in systemic sarcoidosis. The Journal of Experimental Medicine. 2005;**201**:755-767

[37] Rotsinger JE, Celada LJ, Polosukhin VV, Atkinson JB, Drake WP. Molecular analysis of sarcoidosis granulomas reveals antimicrobial targets. American Journal of Respiratory Cell and Molecular Biology. 2016;**55**:128-134

[38] Drake WP, Oswald-Richter K, Richmond BW, et al. Oral antimycobacterial therapy in chronic cutaneous sarcoidosis: A randomized, single-masked, placebo-controlled study. JAMA Dermatology. 2013;**149**:1040-1049

[39] Salin-Pascual RJ, Rosas M, Jimenez-Genchi A, Rivera-Meza BL, Delgado-Parra V. Antidepressant effect of transdermal nicotine patches in nonsmoking patients with major depression. The Journal of Clinical Psychiatry. 1996;**57**:387-389

[40] Ungprasert P, Crowson CS, Matteson EL. Smoking, obesity and risk of sarcoidosis: A population-based nested case-control study. Respiratory Medicine. 2016;**120**:87-90

[41] Newman LS, Rose CS, Bresnitz EA, et al. A case control etiologic study of sarcoidosis: Environmental and occupational risk factors. American Journal of Respiratory and Critical Care Medicine. 2004;**170**:1324-1330

[42] Julian MW, Shao G, Schlesinger LS, et al. Nicotine treatment improves Toll-like receptor 2 and Toll-like receptor 9 responsiveness in active pulmonary sarcoidosis. Chest. 2013;**143**:461-470

[43] Sugano N, Shimida K, Ito K, Murai S. Nicotine inhibits the prodiction of inflammatory mediators in U937 cells through modulation of nuclear factor-kB activation. Biochemal and Biophysical Research Communications. 1998;**252**:25-28

[44] Zheng YS, Wu ZS, Zhang LY, et al. Nicotine ameliorates experimental severe acute pancreatitis via enhancing immunoregulation of CD4+ CD25+ regulatory T cells. Pancreas. 2015;**44**:500-506

[45] Drake WP, Richmond BW, Oswald-Richter K, et al. Effects of broad-spectrum antimycobacterial therapy on chronic pulmonary sarcoidosis. Sarcoidosis Vasc Diffuse Lung Disease. 2014;**30**:201-211

Chapter 3

Mammary Gland Sarcoidosis

Patricia López Arribas, Maria Elena Martínez Gómez and Alvaro Zapico Goñi

Abstract

Sarcoidosis is a benign systemic granulomatous pathology of unknown etiology. Mammary involvement is rare, less than 1% of all cases. That is the reason that makes necessary an optimal differential diagnosis to rule out malignant pathology as the main diagnosis. Imaging tests such as mammography, ultrasound, or MRI contribute to the diagnosis but are unable to establish a certain diagnosis. When a mammary sarcoidosis is suspected by fine needle aspiration cytology, exceptional procedures are necessary to confirm the disease and to exclude a coexisting carcinoma. Malignancy may develop in patients with sarcoidosis, sarcoidosis may develop in patients with breast cancer, the two diseases may develop in tandem, or breast cancer may cause a sarcoidosis-like granulomatous response. Other illnesses that should rule out are granulomatous diseases, which could be differentiated into infectious causes such as tuberculosis and primary inflammatory diseases such as idiopathic granulomatous mastitis. The silicone of gel breast implants may originate a sarcoidosis-like reaction as the result of an acceleration of an already existing hypersensitivity response, resulting in breast sarcoidosis. The management of sarcoidosis in the breast is usually enough with an excisional biopsy. The prognosis of mammary sarcoidosis in not unknown.

Keywords: sarcoidosis, mammary gland, breast, granulomatous mastitis

1. Introduction

Sarcoidosis is a multisystemic granulomatous disease of unknown etiology [1]. Our knowledge of the pathogenesis of sarcoidosis has improved and provided more potential causes of this pathology. Any adjuvant agent of sarcoidosis must be able to cause noncaseating granulomas that are the pathologic hallmark of the disease accompanied by a heterogeneous clinical features [2].

The origin is the failure of the cellular immune response after exposure to an environmental, occupational, or infectious hazard and may affect multiple organs, inclusive breast tissue [3].

Almost 80–90% of patients have lung or hilar lymph nodes affected. These are the most frequent organs involved. Although, the effect on the eyes, skin, nervous system, locomotors system, lacrimal and salivary glands, heart, locomotors system, and kidney in sarcoidosis has also been described [1]. Sarcoid involvement of the mammary gland parenchyma has been extremely infrequent in patients with this pathology, less than 1% of the overall diagnosed patients. African American,

IntechOpen

Afro-Caribbean, Swedish, and Danish individuals are more frequent affected. It is more common in women in their third and fourth decade of life and may often seem to be breast carcinoma [4].

The descriptions of mammary gland sarcoidosis differ from nodules with ill-defined margins or spiculated as observed in malignant tumors, negative imaging, or other nonspecific appearances [3]. The most common symptom is a palpable breast lesion. Because sarcoidosis can mimic breast cancer, it makes the differential diagnosis necessary and not easy [3].

2. Etiology

Sarcoidosis was first described more than 100 years ago, and since then its origin is uncertain, the etiologic determinants causing this disease remain uncertain. The bibliography suggests that host immunologic, genetic, and environmental adjuvants interact together to develop sarcoidosis. The most typical immunological characteristic is noncaseating granulomas, promoting local expression of T helper-1 (and Th17) cytokines and chemokines, dysfunctional regulatory T-cell responses, dysregulated Toll-like receptor signaling, and oligoclonal proliferation of CD4+ T cells consistent with chronic antigenic stimulation. A lot of environmental adjuvants have been proposed to be the origin of sarcoidosis.

Publications of several groups associate mycobacterial or propionibacterial organisms in the etiology of sarcoidosis based on tissue analyses and immunologic responses in sarcoidosis patients. Despite the studies, there is no agreement on the origin of a microbial pathogenesis of sarcoidosis. Others groups postulate that sarcoidosis is caused by an active viable replicating infection, while other groups contend there is no clinical, pathologic, or microbiologic evidence for such a pathogenic mechanism [2]. The authors postulate a new hypothesis that proposes that sarcoidosis is triggered by a hyperimmune Th1 response to pathogenic microbial and tissue antigens associated with the aberrant aggregation of serum amyloid A within granulomas, which promotes chronic granulomatous inflammation with no infection.

3. Clinical manifestations

In the mammary gland, the symptomatology is a breast mass that could be unique or multiple and unilateral or bilateral. Patients do not present infectious or inflammatory symptoms with no effect on the skin. Moreover, the masses are not painful. During the examination it is important not to forget systemic symptoms than can orient our diagnosis because although breast sarcoidosis may be the first affected organ, most of the times the diagnosis is already done.

4. Diagnosis

The symptomatology of sarcoidosis is strongly related to the extent of granulomatous inflammation and the function of the affected organs.

To make a correct diagnosis and establish a correct treatment are very important to assess the impact of sarcoidosis in the organs functions, as well as the impact on quality of life to avoid premature death.

In the mammary gland, the most common symptom is a breast nodule, single or multiple. It is essential to make a differential diagnosis. Starting with the physical examination, usually finding a nontender, firm, and mobile lesion, with a normal nipple. Sometimes it may have axillary lymphadenopathy and other times the mass is fixed, tender, and suggests a carcinoma instead a benign lesion.

Continuing with the study, the next step is the imaging techniques. The first one usually is the mammography that shows a nonspecific, ill-defined lesion with low density, poorly outlined without microcalcifications. There are no definite patterns on ultrasound, so it does not lead to a definitive diagnosis, but we can point out the irregularity of the contours, hypoechoic spiculation, and nonhomogeneous internal echostructure of the nodule (**Figure 1**) [5].

The high-field system MR is complementary to the previous ones. Images can show the nodule to be an isolated signal-intensive inhomogeneous tumor with irregular contours, fast contrast enhancement, and an early "washout" phenomenon often observed in carcinomas or in inflammatory lesions of the breast. Therefore, we must not forget that imaging test does not offer a definitive diagnosis, and we must confirm it with pathological studies.

Also you may rule out infection origin, performing microbiologic test as stains for acid-fast bacilli and fungi.

The pathological study of a biopsy of the breast demonstrates chronic granulomatous inflammatory process, with epithelioid granulomas and non-necrotizing giant cells (**Figure 2**).

Breast sarcoidosis is very rare; generally, a fine needle biopsy is not enough, and an excisional biopsy is necessary to confirm the diagnosis.

The diagnosis is suspected by the typical radiologic manifestations and supported by histologic evidence of noncaseating granulomas in the absence of infection and exclusion of other types of granulomatous affections [6].

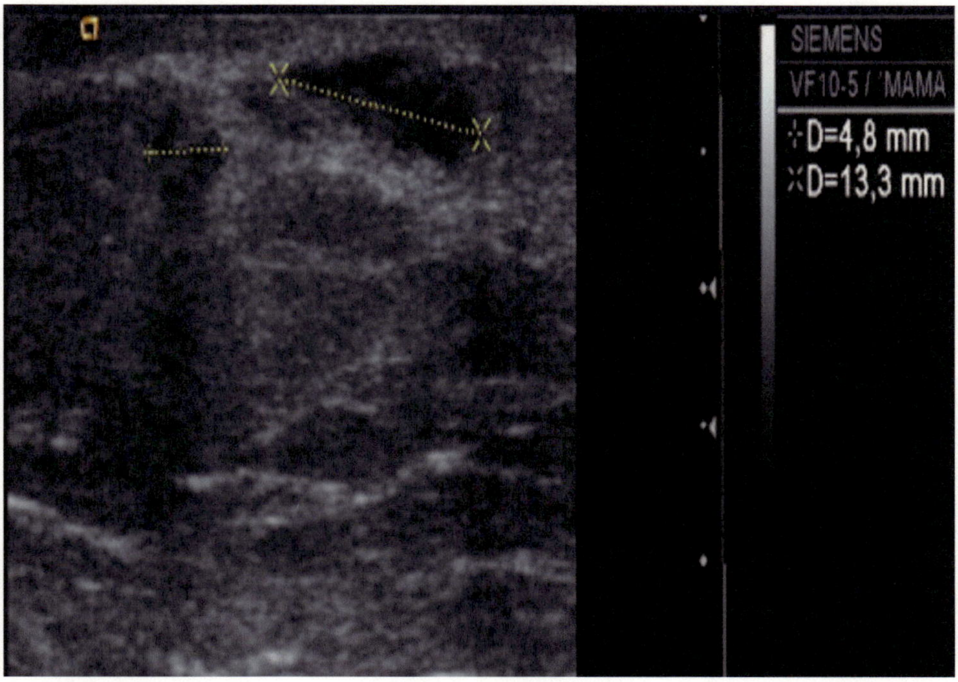

Figure 1.
Ultrasound test with two nonspecific hypoechoic nodules.

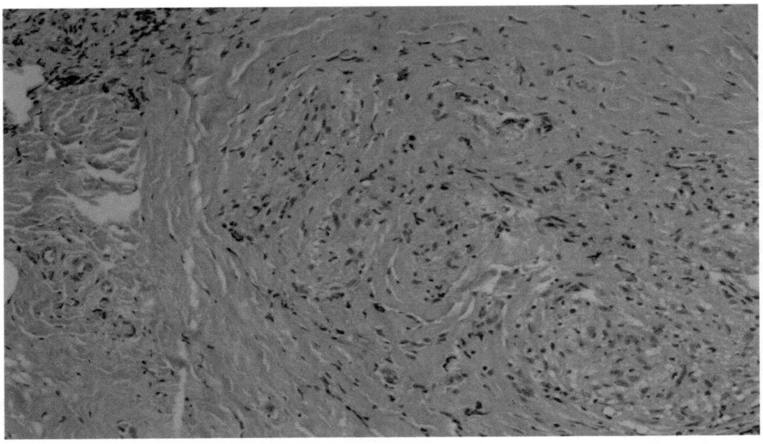

Figure 2.
Chronic granulomatous inflammatory process, with epithelioid granulomas and non-necrotizing giant cells.

5. Differential diagnosis

We should rule out some diseases before the diagnosis of sarcoidosis in the breast (**Table 1**).

5.1 Malignant pathology

The most important and the most frequent is malignant pathology of the breast. The American Cancer Society (ACS) estimates that almost 300,000 women will receive

Neoplasia	Benign	Fibroadenoma
		Cyst
		Fibrocystic changes
		Galactocele
		Breast abscess
		Radial scar
		Fat necrosis
		Fibrosis
		Diabetic mastopathy
	Malignant	Invasive carcinoma
		Breast lymphoma
		Metastasis
Granulomatous disease	Infectious causes	Tuberculosis
		Fungal infections
		Actinomycosis
		Histoplasmosis
	Inflammatory diseases	Wegener's granulomatosis
		Idiopathic granulomatous mastitis

Table 1.
Differential diagnosis of breast sarcoidosis.

a diagnosis of malignant breast per year. A breast mass is suspicious until proven otherwise. The first step is imaging test such as mammography, ultrasound, and MRI.

As we have described, there are no pathognomonic patterns in the imaging test for sarcoidosis in mammary gland, and it is the same with breast cancer.

Thus, we need to confirm the diagnosis after those techniques; we should perform pathological test and immunohistochemistry to confirm the definitive diagnosis, prognosis criterion, and treatment.

5.2 Idiopathic granulomatous mastitis (IGM)

Idiopathic granulomatous mastitis is an infrequent, chronic, and benign breast pathology, which may imitate mammary gland abscess, cancer, or other granulomatous diseases. Most patients present in the third or fourth decade of life, and it typically is seen in women of childbearing potential from 6 months to 6 years postpartum. It is a diagnosis of exclusion and requires a high index of suspicion [7, 8].

Usually the first diagnose is bacterial mastitis, scheduling multiple antibiotic regimens. When those treatments are not successful, an inflammatory breast cancer is suspected, thus no healing breast nodules. Imaging test and fine needle biopsy for pathological study are not enough to confirm the diagnosis, and an excisional biopsy is mandatory.

Idiopathic granulomatous mastitis is an exclusion diagnosis. Made after demonstration of granulomatous inflammation on mammary gland biopsy and excluding other granulomatous diseases, such as tuberculosis and sarcoidosis.

In sarcoidosis, the most frequent affectation is lung disease (90%), that is why when you suspect a granulomatous disease, you need to rule out this pathology with a chest X-ray, which confirms that no presence of hilar lymphadenopathy [8].

Many cases do not need any treatment and resolve themselves. When an extensive breast affectation exists for a long time with no clinical improvement, other treatments are necessary such as methotrexate, corticosteroids, or surgical excision.

5.3 Tuberculosis

Breast tuberculosis is a pathology characterized by the presence of granulomas. This disease is unusual in Europe, it only presents 0.1% of all mammary gland tumors, but in endemic areas, it increases until 4.5%. Is necessary to rule out other breast pathologies such as abscess, sarcoidosis, idiopathic granulomatous mastitis, or a malignant lesion.

Risk factors for the development of breast TB include lactation, multiparty, immunosuppression, and previous exposure to TB [9, 10].

Usually the main symptom is a single mass; with minor infection or inflammation than in other infectious mastitis. Diagnosis of breast tuberculosis is not easy. Most of the times multiple clinic consultations and tissue biopsies are necessary, Ziehl-Neelsen stain and QuantiFERON-TB Gold test should be performed to help differentiate between breast sarcoidosis and tuberculosis. That is the reason why the treatment is delayed [11].

5.4 Sarcoidosis-like reaction

An event known as autoimmune/inflammatory syndrome triggered by adjuvants might be caused by the combination of silicone implants and sarcoidosis-like reaction with a strange body granulomatous response. Silicone acts as an immunologic adjuvant to generate antigen-specific immune response that causes the proliferation and activation of B and T cells [12].

There are others cases published in the bibliography that report this type of reaction, it may appear in the breast skin, subcutaneous tissue, axillary lymph nodes, and brain, spinal cord, or digestive tract. The pathophysiological mechanism remains unclear. The first hypothesis is a direct granulomatous reaction against silicon particles following extensive systemic dissemination. Finding local granulomatous reaction to silicone after implant rupture and systemic dissemination of silicone gel. The other hypothesis is a full-blown sarcoidosis triggered by silicon as an external adjuvant, in a predisposed patient, which could be included in the context of an autoimmune syndrome induced by adjuvant [13].

5.5 Sarcoidosis mimicking metastatic breast cancer

Sarcoidosis commonly affects the lungs; however, any organ can be involved.

In patients with a history of a malignant disease, when an abnormal nodule is observed in imaging studies, the tendency is to suspect a metastatic lesion. Some studies suggest an increased incidence of sarcoidosis in the event of malignancy and its treatment. Malignancy itself is immunosuppressant; chemotherapy might downregulate sarcoidosis [14, 15]. In addition, an infection acquired during chemotherapy might lead to a sarcoidosis activation.

Other authors propose that a tumor antigen(s) might be the triggering and oligoclonal T-cell hyper-reactivity toward granulomatous disease.

6. Treatment

The treatment of mammary gland sarcoidosis is usually the same as systemic sarcoidosis. To confirm the diagnosis, most of the times, we need an excisional biopsy. When there are no other symptoms, systemic treatment is not necessary.

Conflict of interest

The authors declare no conflict of interest.

Author details

Patricia López Arribas*, Maria Elena Martínez Gómez and Alvaro Zapico Goñi
Hospital Universitario Príncipe de Asturias, Madrid, Spain

*Address all correspondence to: patricialopezar@gmail.com

References

[1] Takahasi R, Shibuya Y, Shijubo N, Asaishi K, Abe S. Mammary involvement in patient with sarcoidosis. Internal Medicine. 2001;**40**:769-771

[2] Chen ES, Moller DR. Etiology of sarcoidosis. Clinics in Chest Medicine. 2008;**29**:365-377

[3] Chen J, Carter R 3rd, Maoz D, Tobar A, Sharon E, Greif F. Breast cancer and sarcoidosis: Case series and review of the literature. Breast Care (Basel). 2015;**10**:137-140

[4] Nicholson BT, Mills SE. Sarcoidosis of the breast: An unusual presentation of a systemic disease. The Breast Journal. 2007;**13**:99-100

[5] Endlich JL, Souza JA, Cynthia A, Osório BT, Lopes Pinto CA, Faria EP, et al. Breast sarcoidosis as the first manifestation of the disease. Breast Journal. 2019;**00**:1-2

[6] Kenzel PP, Hadijuana J, Hosten N, Minguillon C, Oellinger H, Siewert C, et al. Boeck, sarcoidosis of the breast, ultra-sound, and MRI findings. Journal of Computer Assisted Tomography. 1997;**21**:439-441

[7] Poovamma CU, Pais VA, Dolas SC, Prema M, Khandelwal R, Nis-heena R. Idiopathic granulomatous mastitis: A rare entity with a variable presentation. Breast Disease. 2014;**34**:101

[8] Haitz K, Ly A, Smith G. Idiopathic granulomatous mastitis. Cutis. 2019; **103**(1):38-42

[9] Mehta G, Mittal A, Verma S. Breast tuberculosis—Clinical spectrum and management. Indian Journal of Surgery. 2010;**72**(6):433-437

[10] Thimmappa D, Mallikarjuna MN, Vijayakumar A. Breast tuberculosis. Indian Journal of Surgery. 2015;**77**(3): S1378-SS138

[11] Reis J, Boavida J, Bahrami N, Lyngra M, Geitung JT. Breast sarcoidosis: Clinical features, imaging, and histological findings. The Breast Journal. 2021;**27**:44-47

[12] Shoenfeld Y, Agmon-Levin N. ASIA: Autoimmune/inflammatory syndrome induced by adjuvants. Journal of Autoimmunity. 2011;**36**:4-8

[13] Segal Y, Dahan S, Sharif K, Bragazzi NL, Watad A, Amital H. The value of Autoimmune Syndrome Induced by Adjuvant (ASIA) - Shedding light on orphan diseases in autoimmunity. Autoimmunity Reviews. 2018;**5**(17):440-448

[14] Arish N, Kuint R, Sapir E, Levy L, Abutbul A, Fridlender Z, et al. Characteristics of sarcoidosis in patients with previous malignancy: Causality or coincidence? Respiration. 2017;**93**(4):247-252

[15] Bassler R, Birke F. Histopathology of tumor associated sarcoid- like stromal reaction in breast cancer: An analysis of 5 cases with immunohistochemical investigations. Virchows Archiv. A, Pathological Anatomy and Histopathology. 1988;**412**:231-239

Chapter 4

Skeletal Sarcoidosis

Henco Nel and Eli Gabbay

Abstract

Osseous sarcoidosis is an uncommon manifestation, reported in 3–13% of patients with sarcoidosis. Although older literature suggested that hands and feet are most commonly affected, axial bone involvement may be more common than previously reported, since earlier studies relied mostly on plain X-rays, which may be less sensitive for axial bone lesions. Newer imaging modalities such as MRI and PET/CT scanning have demonstrated a larger incidence of vertebral involvement. Bone lesions are commonly asymptomatic and patients who have bone involvement may have higher incidences of multi-organ involvement. Osseous sarcoidosis appears to be mainly osteolytic in nature, but the radiographic appearance may be indistinguishable from other osteolytic lesions and therefore a biopsy is usually required to confirm the diagnosis. The histological findings of sarcoidosis in the bone are the same as in other tissues of the body. No general consensus exists for the treatment of bone sarcoidosis but corticosteroids are the most commonly prescribed first-line drugs. Methotrexate is the most widely studied steroid-sparing agent for sarcoidosis and it has been reported useful for a variety of organ symptoms, but especially where there is bone involvement.

Keywords: osteolytic lesions, vertebral involvement, PET/CT, corticosteroids, methotrexate

1. Introduction

Bone involvement is reported in approximately 3–13% of patients with sarcoidosis [1]. However, its frequency is likely underestimated as it is often asymptomatic [2–4]. The pathogenesis of sarcoidosis involving the skeletal system remains unknown. Patients with skeletal sarcoidosis usually have multiple bones involved and numerous other extra-osseous manifestations [3, 5]. Newer imaging modalities have demonstrated a relative increase in axial involvement [3, 4]. Treatment guidelines for skeletal sarcoidosis are lacking and evidence comes primarily from retrospective case series and individual case reports [3, 4]. Nonetheless, most patients with bone involvement respond well to corticosteroids in combination with methotrexate [5].

2. Pathophysiology

The pathogenesis of sarcoidosis specifically involving bone is unclear. Some authors have postulated that antigenic particles are spread hematogenously or through the lymphatic system, creating granulomas within the bone, bone marrow, and other organs [4]. This hypothesis may help to explain the greater frequency of liver, spleen, and extrathoracic lymph node involvement in patients with bone sarcoidosis [4]. The mechanisms of osteolysis in sarcoidosis also remain unclear. Mechanisms that have been postulated include: high levels of 1,25 $(OH)_2$ D3 activity stimulating osteoclastic activity, local granuloma-induced osteoclastic reaction and the sarcoid granuloma being a source of an osteoclastic activating factor inducing bone resorption. However, none of these hypotheses have been shown to provide a satisfactory explanation related to the presence of bone lesions in sarcoidosis [1].

3. Epidemiology

Bone involvement is reported in 3–13% of patients with sarcoidosis, although its frequency is likely to be underestimated as it is often asymptomatic [1–3]. Imaging modalities such as magnetic resonance imaging (MRI) or positron emission tomography (PET)/computed tomography (CT) scans appear to identify more patients with bone involvement than historically appreciated using conventional radiography [6]. However, these imaging modalities are not routinely used for the diagnosis of skeletal sarcoidosis and are usually used to characterize organ involvement in systemic sarcoidosis or for the investigation of suspected cancer or fever of unknown origin [3, 4, 6]. Skeletal sarcoidosis appears to be more common in middle-aged and elderly white women [3, 4]. Zhou and colleagues demonstrated that white patients were three times more likely than blacks to have bone sarcoidosis while another study of 20 patients with bone sarcoidosis reported that 95% of these patients were white. Although this difference may reflect demographic characteristics at their institutions, it raises the possibility of a racial predilection [3, 4].

4. Clinical manifestations

Patients with bone sarcoidosis usually have numerous other extra-osseous manifestations and compared to matched cases, bone sarcoidosis patients have more multi-organ involvement than controls [3–5]. Patients with skeletal sarcoidosis also typically have more than one bone involved [3]. However, osseous involvement is frequently asymptomatic and can be incidentally detected in up to half of the patients [3, 5].

Skeletal sarcoidosis can involve focal areas of both the appendicular and axial skeleton. Pain and swelling are the most common symptoms [1, 3]. Older studies found that the hands and feet are most commonly affected, with axial bone involvement rarely reported [1]. However, axial bone involvement may be more common than previously reported, since earlier studies relied mostly on plain X-rays, which may be less sensitive for axial bone lesions [4]. Newer imaging modalities such as MRI and PET/CT scanning have demonstrated a larger incidence of vertebral involvement, and a recent retrospective study demonstrated that up to 70 percent of patients with skeletal sarcoidosis may have spinal disease [4].

4.1 Axial involvement

Axial sarcoidosis most commonly affects the spine followed by the pelvis [3–5]. Vertebral involvement is mostly asymptomatic and underdiagnosed [3]. The disease frequently affects the lower thoracic and upper lumbar vertebrae, but the cervical spine including the atlantoaxial (C1-C2) joint may also be involved [7, 8]. In symptomatic patients, pain is a prominent feature, especially at the thoracolumbar region [4]. With the more frequent use of advanced imaging (MRI, PET/CT) to evaluate sarcoidosis, there has been increasing recognition of the greater relative frequency of axial involvement. In one series of 20 patients with osseous sarcoid, involvement of the axial skeleton, especially the pelvis and lumbar spine, was seen in 90 percent of patients but was often asymptomatic [3]. In another study, 3.5 percent of patients (64 out of 1802) with sarcoidosis had bone involvement and axial involvement was more common than appendicular involvement [4]. Skull sarcoidosis is uncommon and a recent systematic review yielded only 22 known cases, all of which were case reports [9]. In 35% of these cases, skull sarcoidosis was detected incidentally in asymptomatic patients [9].

4.2 Appendicular involvement

The most commonly affected appendicular skeletal sites are the proximal and middle phalanges of the hands [1]. With phalangeal involvement, patients can experience local pain and tenderness in the affected region, which can exhibit swelling, reduced function, distortion of fingers, and overlying erythema [3, 5]. The findings are often bilateral but asymmetric [1, 3]. There is also frequent involvement of the feet [3, 4]. Hand lesions were more common in African Americans in one study, but bone involvement overall was more frequent in whites [4].

5. Laboratory findings

Laboratory findings in bone sarcoidosis are generally nonspecific and similar to those seen in other forms of systemic sarcoidosis without bone disease [4, 10]. However, bone marrow involvement may cause leukopenia [11] and one study showed a significantly lower white blood cell (WBC) count in patients with skeletal sarcoidosis, compared to sarcoidosis patients without bone involvement [4].

Erythrocyte sedimentation rate (ESR), alkaline phosphatase (ALP), and serum calcium are normal in the majority of patients with skeletal sarcoidosis and this may reflect a distinct pathophysiology compared to other diseases that affect bones, such as Paget's disease, malignancy, osteoporosis, or osteomalacia [3]. Therefore, skeletal sarcoidosis should be considered in sarcoidosis patients who present with spinal and pelvic bone lesions, especially among asymptomatic patients with normal serum calcium and (ALP) [3].

6. Imaging

A number of changes can be seen using conventional radiographs, MRI, and PET/CT in patients with osseous sarcoidosis [4]. Conventional radiographs are usually sufficient for evaluation of the hands and feet, but MRI and PET/CT are more sensitive for the detection of changes in other parts of the skeleton [4].

6.1 Conventional (plain) radiography

A plain radiograph cannot reliably reflect early bone lesions, only the gross changes are clear [12]. Nonetheless, conventional radiography can be used to reveal the location of sarcoid bone lesions in the small bones of the hands and feet [10]. Classic sarcoid lesions in the small bones of the hands and feet are well characterized and diagnosed with conventional radiographs, on which they demonstrate the familiar "lacy" lytic appearance. The resulting alignment deformities in the hands and feet are often due to pathologic fractures with bone collapse rather than joint abnormalities [13]. Although osseous sarcoidosis appears to be mainly osteolytic in nature, osteoblastic lesions have also been reported [12]. Sclerotic changes may represent the result of a secondary reaction related to treatment and they are not necessarily lesions that have been osteoblastic from the beginning [12].

Other radiographic bone lesions that have been described include diffuse marrow infiltration, punched-out lesions, permeative lesions and destructive lesions (dactylitis). Diffuse marrow infiltration with absorption and disruption of bone trabeculae is more frequently, earlier and accurately identified by bone scan than plain radiography. Punched-out lesions are small cortical defects surrounded by normal bone, usually seen in relatively unaggressive sarcoidosis, and persist indefinitely. Permeative lesions start with tunneling in the cortex of the shafts of small bones, followed by remodeling of the cortical and trabecular architecture to give a reticular pattern. Destructive lesions include rapidly advancing bone involvement with multiple fractures, devitalized cortex, considerable soft tissue swelling, but no periosteal reaction such as new bone formation. Destructive lesions are rare and seen in <0.2% of cases. More than seventy percent of patients can have a combination of lesions [12].

6.2 Radionuclide bone scan

Radionuclide scans appear to pick up the infiltration of sarcoidosis earlier and more accurately than radiographs and they successfully demonstrate up to 30% more osseous lesions than conventional radiography [12]. However, sarcoidosis bone lesions show variable uptake on bone scintigraphy and lesions that are occult on technetium-99 m (Tc99m) can demonstrate mild to marked fluorodeoxyglucose (FDG) avidity on PET/CT throughout the axial and appendicular skeleton [3].

6.3 PET/CT

A systematic review of the utility of PET imaging to monitor sarcoidosis disease activity noted that PET may often detect incidental lesions [14]. However, it is currently unclear how often asymptomatic osseous lesions might be incidentally detected with PET imaging in sarcoidosis [3]. PET scans in patients with skeletal sarcoidosis typically show active metabolism in bone, but no feature can reliably distinguish sarcoidosis from malignant lesions, particularly in the spine and pelvis and bone biopsies may be required to exclude malignancy [5]. A study from the Netherlands of 122 patients with biopsy-proven severe sarcoidosis (defined as persistent, unexplained disease-related disabling symptoms) revealed focal bone uptake and/or more diffuse bone marrow involvement in more than one-third of patients by use of PET/CT scanning, although 94 percent of the lesions were not evident on low-dose bone CT [6]. This was much higher than expected according to most previous published studies. Moreover, it showed that PET/CT may be an excellent modality to detect bone involvement compared with more conventional modalities [2, 15]. Also of great interest was the low rate of abnormalities on low-dose CT. Clear bone lesions on CT were identified in only 2 of the 32 patients with PET-detected bone abnormalities. This finding suggests that physiological changes may precede morphologic changes [6].

The use of PET to assess the extent of disease can also uncover a suitable location for biopsy to obtain histological evidence for the diagnosis [6]. Furthermore, assessment of inflammatory activity is helpful to monitor the course of the disease and guide therapeutic strategies, but establishing the presence of inflammatory activity can be a challenge for clinicians. In recent years, PET has been shown to be a very sensitive technique to assess the inflammatory activity in sarcoidosis by detecting and quantifying the level of inflammatory and granulomatous reactions that occur in the lungs and elsewhere in the body [16, 17]. Several reports have demonstrated a significant reduction of FDG uptake after the initiation of treatment in bone sarcoidosis patients [3, 6, 18]. An example of a pretreatment and posttreatment PET scan of a patient with widespread bone sarcoidosis is shown in **Figure 1**.

6.4 MRI

MRI may be the most sensitive modality in the detection of axial skeleton, large tubular bones and bone marrow involvement in sarcoidosis. Long bone and axial skeletal involvement may be occult at conventional radiography but depicted at MR imaging, with an appearance that resembles that of osseous metastases [13]. With the majority of large tubular bone lesions, there is no MRI evidence of periosteal involvement or cortical destruction, although cortical disruption and extraosseous extension are usually seen when small bones are involved. The lack of cortical destruction with large-bone lesions might explain why the majority of these lesions are radiographically occult and clinically silent. On MRI, granulomatous infiltration

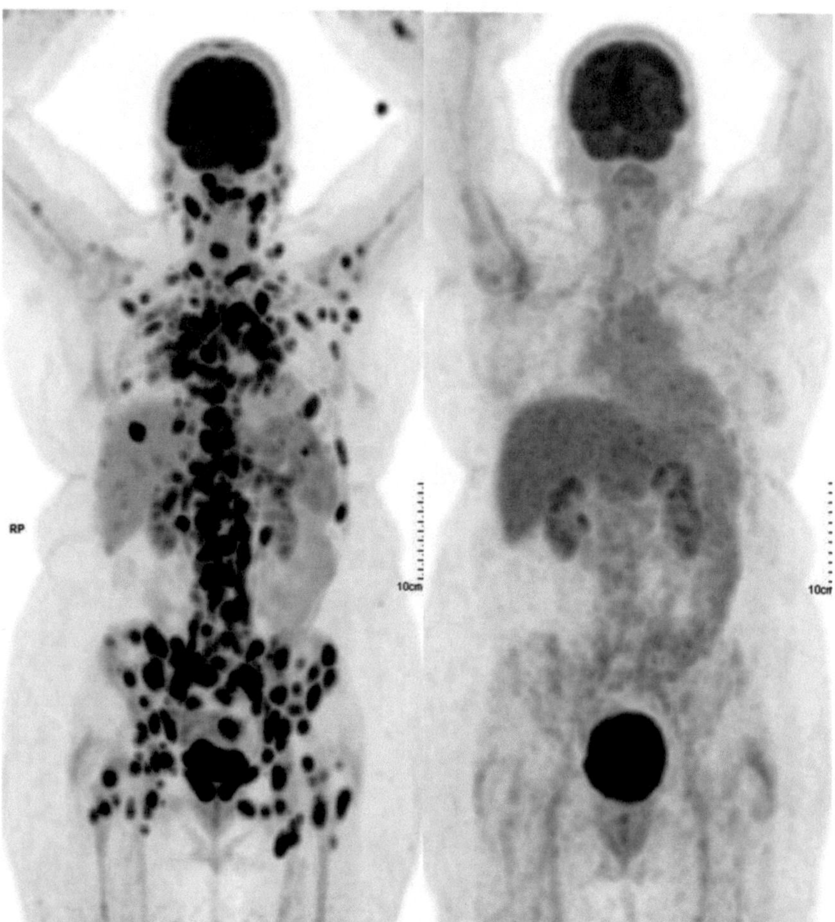

Figure 1.
PET/CT scan showing marked improvement after initiation of immunosuppressive therapy with no definitive evidence for residual FDG-avid disease (Right), compared to previously demonstrated intense FDG-uptake within the lymph nodes above and below the diaphragm, within multiple skeletal lesions and within lesions involving the lungs, liver and spleen (Left).

of the bone marrow results in an abnormal signal. The lesions are most often hypointense on T1-weighted imaging, hyperintense on T2-weighted and Short Tau Inversion Recovery (STIR) imaging and show enhancement after contrast administration [13]. **Figure 2** demonstrates contrast enhancing lesions of the skull and C2 vertebra.

Despite the sensitivity of MRI compared with conventional radiography, osseous sarcoidosis lesions cannot be reliably distinguished from metastatic lesions on routine MRI [19]. In a comparison of osseous sarcoidosis with osseous metastatic lesions, the presence of intra- or perilesional fat, lesional border characteristics (i.e., sharply defined, brush-like, or poorly defined), and the presence of an extraosseous soft tissue mass, as well as posterior element involvement of spinal changes, were indicative of osseous sarcoidosis, but overall had only moderate sensitivity for the diagnosis, despite relatively high specificity [19].

MR imaging of sarcoidosis lesions of the small bones also provides information not available at radiography, demonstrating marrow lesions that are radiographically occult, extension of granulomas beyond the cortex, and periosseous soft-tissue involvement [13]. Large bone lesions can have a variety of appearances,

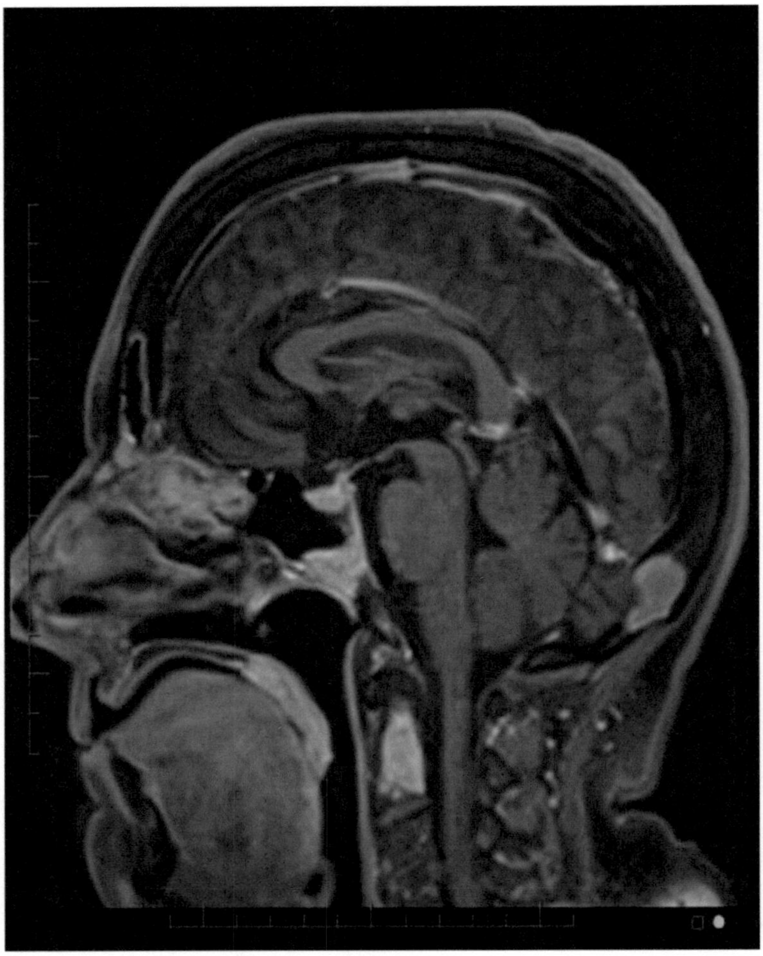

Figure 2.
Post-contrast T1 weighted SPACE sequence with fat saturation demonstrates contrast enhancement of osseous lesions of the clivus, occipital bone, and C2 vertebra. MRI demonstrates the C2 lesion involves the vertebral body and odontoid process.

including round, cannonball-like intramedullary lesions, confluent irregular marrow infiltration, less well-defined discrete lesions with a "starry sky" appearance, and patchy, diffuse intramedullary lesions [13].

6.5 CT scan

Computed tomography (CT) scanning is often used to evaluate pulmonary or lymph node involvement in sarcoidosis, and bony lesions can be detected on these scans. However, CT scan is nonspecific, as is conventional radiography, and the sensitivity of CT for osseous sarcoid is lower than MRI or PET/CT [4]. On radiography and CT, sarcoidosis bone lesions can be mixed, lytic, or sclerotic but may also be undetectable, particularly in the axial skeleton and long bones [19].

7. Pathology

The histological findings of sarcoidosis in the bone are the same as in other tissues of the body [12]. The lesion of sarcoidosis is a focal, well-defined granuloma formed by the accumulation of epithelial cells, multinucleated giant cells, lymphocytes, macrophages and fibroblasts. The centre of the granuloma is composed of macrophage-derived cells and CD4+ T cells, whereas the periphery of the granuloma is composed of a large number of antigen-presenting interdigitating macrophages, CD4+ and CD8+ T cells [20, 21]. **Figure 3** demonstrates a cluster of well-formed, non-necrotising granulomas.

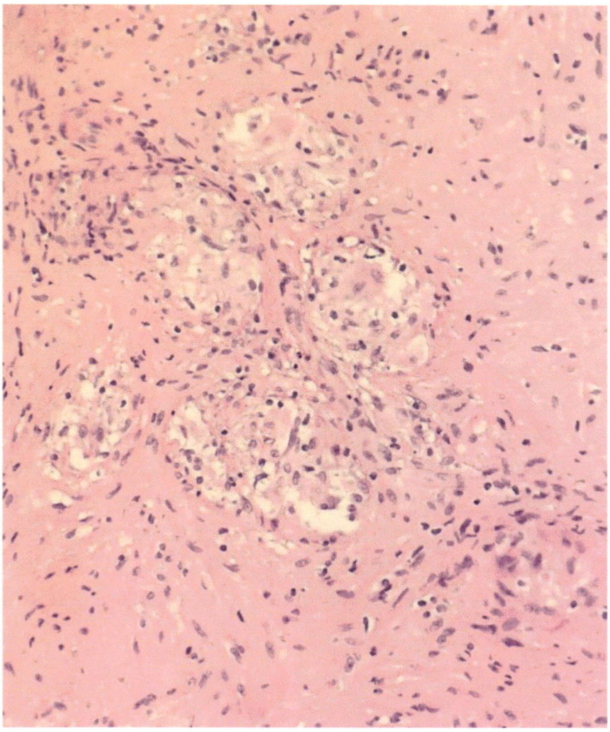

Figure 3.
Microscopic examination of clivus bone tissue demonstrating a cluster of well-formed, non-necrotising granulomas.

8. Diagnosis

In patients with classic skeletal lesions, either on conventional hand radiographs or with characteristic lesions detected on MRI or PET/CT, and biopsy-proven sarcoidosis in another organ, a biopsy may not be necessary, depending upon the clinical context [1, 13]. In one study, non-caseating granulomas were identified in all thirty-five patients with a positive MRI or PET/CT who underwent bone biopsy [3]. This observation might suggest that pathological confirmation may not be required for patients with typical imaging patterns [5].

However, because it is not possible to reliably distinguish granulomatous bone involvement of sarcoidosis from other causes by MRI or other imaging modalities, a biopsy is often required [4, 19]. A site appropriate for biopsy should be readily identified and this should be guided by imaging and symptoms [4]. In those without a prior diagnosis of sarcoidosis, radiologists should include sarcoidosis in the differential diagnosis of musculoskeletal disease detected on MRI in the appropriate clinical setting and should be alerted that large bone and axial skeleton sarcoidosis lesions encountered on MRI might resemble metastatic lesions [22, 23].

9. Differential diagnosis

Despite the increased sensitivity of MRI and PET/CT scans compared to conventional radiography, no imaging modality can reliably distinguish the features of osseous sarcoidosis and other skeletal pathologies [5, 6, 19].

Major conditions that should be considered in the differential diagnosis of bone sarcoidosis include:

Metastatic cancer or hematopoietic malignancy – The bone lesions in sarcoidosis can mimic those of metastatic cancer (eg, of the breast or prostate), lymphoma, multiple myeloma, or osseous hemangioma [19, 24, 25]. In patients with sarcoidosis documented in other organs and tissues and without any evidence of malignancy, it may be possible to infer that bone lesions, particularly with characteristic imaging changes, are due to sarcoidosis rather than malignancy. However, malignancy and sarcoidosis cannot be reliably distinguished on plain radiographs, by MRI [19], or on PET/CT. Therefore, a biopsy is often required to make this distinction if there is any clinical uncertainty [6].

Infection – Disseminated granulomatous infections like tuberculosis can result in focal or multifocal bone lesions. Fungal infections including disseminated cryptococcosis can also cause widespread osteolytic lesions and should be considered, particularly in immunosuppressed patients [26]. Serologic testing and/or biopsy and culture of the affected area can be performed to exclude infection [27].

Paget's disease of bone – Sarcoidosis of the long bones may resemble Paget's disease since both disorders are associated with increased uptake on bone scans and with lytic and sclerotic lesions on radiography. Unlike Paget's disease, however, the serum alkaline phosphatase (ALP) concentration is usually normal in patients with sarcoidosis [3].

10. Treatment

Treatment guidelines for extrapulmonary sarcoidosis are lacking and evidence for benefit in patients with osseous sarcoidosis comes primarily from retrospective case series and individual case reports [3, 4]. Most patients with osseous sarcoidosis will already be receiving treatment for other disease manifestations when bone disease is identified or will require therapy for these manifestations if they are newly diagnosed [3, 4]. Isolated, asymptomatic bone disease may not require systemic immunosuppressive treatment and some cases of spontaneous remission have been reported [28, 29]. Nevertheless, corticosteroids remain the most commonly prescribed first-line therapy for bone sarcoidosis. Corticosteroids have been shown to be very effective in providing symptomatic relief and treatment with these agents may also result in radiological improvement [5, 30]. However, some patients may have persistent radiological abnormalities despite clinical resolution [30].

Prolonged corticosteroid therapy is associated with long-term complications and methotrexate or hydroxychloroquine have often been used, usually in combination with corticosteroids, in order to allow lower corticosteroid dose [4]. Methotrexate is the most widely studied steroid-sparing agent for sarcoidosis and it has been reported useful for a variety of organ symptoms but especially where there is bone involvement [4, 28]. Most patients with bone sarcoidosis respond well to corticosteroids in combination with methotrexate [5]. **Figure 1** demonstrates the radiological improvement in a patient that received prednisolone and methotrexate. Other second line-agents including azathioprine and third-line treatments such as anti-TNF inhibitors are often prescribed for patients with severe sarcoidosis, whose disease cannot be controlled by low-dose corticosteroids and may represent alternative options, although these are not well studied in bone sarcoidosis [4]. However, there is evidence that tumor necrosis factor (TNF) is involved in the pathogenesis of sarcoidosis, and there have been reports of successful treatment of refractory bone sarcoidosis with anti-TNF agents [3, 4]. In rare cases with irreversible bone pain, neurological involvement, or pathological fractures, surgery can be considered [30].

11. Prognosis

The presence of bone lesions generally implies a more advanced, chronic, and severe disorder overall, with more organs and tissues affected by sarcoidosis [2, 15]. Nevertheless, most patients with bone sarcoidosis respond well to corticosteroids in combination with methotrexate and this usually results in symptomatic improvement [4, 5]. Infrequently, spontaneous remission of skeletal sarcoidosis may also occur [29].

12. Conclusion

The incidence of skeletal sarcoidosis is probably underestimated as it is often asymptomatic. However, bone involvement in patients with sarcoidosis generally implies multi-organ and chronic disease. Skeletal sarcoidosis appears to be more common in middle-aged and elderly white women and frequently involves the spine. Laboratory findings are generally nonspecific and similar to those seen in other forms of systemic sarcoidosis without bone involvement. Conventional radiographs are usually sufficient for evaluation of the hands and feet, but MRI and PET/CT are more sensitive for the detection of changes in other parts of the skeleton. Newer imaging modalities are increasingly being used to evaluate skeletal involvement in sarcoidosis but most patients still require a biopsy to confirm the diagnosis. Although no general consensus exists for the management of bone sarcoidosis, the majority of patients respond well to corticosteroids in combination with methotrexate.

Acknowledgements

Jack Bendat and the Bendat Respiratory Research and Development Fund at St John of God Hospital Subiaco.

Author details

Henco Nel[1]* and Eli Gabbay[2]

1 Sir Charles Gairdner Hospital, Nedlands, Australia

2 School of Medicine, University of Notre Dame, Fremantle, Australia

*Address all correspondence to: henco.nel@health.wa.gov.au

References

[1] Wilcox A, Bharadwaj P, Sharma OP. Bone sarcoidosis. Curr Opin Rheumatol 2000; 12:321.

[2] James DG, Neville E, Carstairs LS. Bone and joint sarcoidosis. Semin Arthritis Rheum 1976; 6:53.

[3] Sparks JA, McSparron JI, Shah N, et al. Osseous sarcoidosis: clinical characteristics, treatment, and outcomes--experience from a large, academic hospital. Semin Arthritis Rheum 2014; 44:371.

[4] Zhou Y, Lower EE, Li H, et al. Clinical characteristics of patients with bone sarcoidosis. Semin Arthritis Rheum 2017; 47:143.

[5] Ben Hassine I, Rein C, Comarmond C, et al. Osseous sarcoidosis: A multicenter retrospective case-control study of 48 patients. Joint Bone Spine 2019; 86(6):789-793.

[6] Mostard RL, Prompers L, Weijers RE, et al. F-18 FDG PET/CT for detecting bone and bone marrow involvement in sarcoidosis patients. Clin Nucl Med 2012; 37:21.

[7] Cutler SS, Sankaranarayanan G. Vertebral sarcoidosis. JAMA 1978; 240:557.

[8] Sundaram M, Place H, Shaffer WO, Martin DS. Progressive destructive vertebral sarcoid leading to surgical fusion. Skeletal Radiol 1999; 28:717.

[9] Robles LA, Matilla AF, Covarrubias MP. Sarcoidosis of the Skull: A Systematic Review. World neurosurgery 2020; 139:387-394.

[10] Kuzyshyn, H, Feinstein, D, Kolasinski, SL, et al. Osseous sarcoidosis: a case series. Rheumatol Int. 2015; 35: 925-933.

[11] Yanardağ H, Pamuk GE, Karayel T, Demirci S. Bone marrow involvement in sarcoidosis: an analysis of 50 bone marrow samples. Haematologia (Budap). 2002;32(4):419-425.

[12] Yaghmai I. Radiographic, angiographic and radionuclide manifestations of osseous sarcoidosis. Radiographics 1983;3(3):375-396.

[13] Moore SL, Teirstein AE. Musculoskeletal sarcoidosis: spectrum of appearances at MR imaging. Radiographics 2003;23(6):1389-1399.

[14] Treglia G, Taralli S, Giordano A. Emerging role of whole-body 18F-fluorodeoxyglucose positron emission tomography as a marker of disease activity in patients with sarcoidosis: a systematic review. Sarcoidosis Vasc Diffuse Lung Dis 2011; 28:87-94.

[15] Neville E, Carstairs LS, James DG. Sarcoidosis of bone. Q J Med 1977; 46:215.

[16] Teirstein AS, Machac J, Almeida O, et al. Results of 188 whole-body fluorodeoxyglucose positron emission tomography scans in 137 patients with sarcoidosis. Chest 2007; 132:1949 – 1953.

[17] Braun JJ, Kessler R, Constantinesco A, Imperiale A. 18F-FDG PET/CT in sarcoidosis management: review and report of 20 cases. Eur J Nucl Med Mol Imaging 2008; 35:1537 – 1543.

[18] Nel H, Davis B, Adler B, Gabbay E. Case report of osteolytic lesions in a patient with multisystem granulomatous disease. BMJ Case Rep. 2021;14(6):e242685.

[19] Moore SL, Kransdorf MJ, Schweitzer ME, et al. Can sarcoidosis and metastatic bone lesions be reliably

differentiated on routine MRI? AJR Am J Roentgenol 2012; 198:1387.

[20] Semenzato G, Pezzutto A, Chilosi M, Pizzolo G.Redistribution of T lymphocytes in the lymph nodes of patients with sarcoidosis. N Engl J Med 1982; 306(1):48-49.

[21] Kasahara K, Kobayashi K, Shikama Y, et al. The role of monokines in granuloma formation in mice: the ability of interleukin 1 and tumor necrosis factor-alpha to induce lung granulomas. Clin Immunol Immunopathol 1989; 51(3):419-425.

[22] Talmi D, Smith S, Mulligan ME. Central skeletal sarcoidosis mimicking metastatic disease. Skeletal Radiol 2008; 37(8):757-761.

[23] Waanders F, van Hengel P, Krikke A, et al. Sarcoidosis mimicking metastatic disease: a case report and review of the literature. Neth J Med 2006; 64(9):342-345.

[24] Vinnicombe S, Heron C, Wansbrough-Jones M. Dense bones. Br J Radiol 1992; 65:1049.

[25] Sun SS, Tsai SC, Hung CJ, et al. Tc-99m MDP and Ga-67 citrate scintigraphic findings in sarcoidosis with osseous involvement. Clin Nucl Med 2001; 26:472.

[26] Yang CJ, Hwang JJ, Wang TH, et al. Clinical and radiographic presentations of pulmonary cryptococcosis in immunocompetent patients. Scand J Infect Dis 2006; 38:788.

[27] Kenney CM 3rd, Goldstein SJ. MRI of sarcoid spondylodiskitis. J Comput Assist Tomogr 1992; 16:660.

[28] Sweiss NJ, Lower EE, Korsten P, et al. Bone Health Issues in Sarcoidosis. Current Rheumatology Reports 2011;13(3):265-272.

[29] Salmon JH, Perotin JM, Direz G, et al. Vertebral sarcoidosis. Spontaneous favorable outcome: A case report and literature review. Rev Med Interne 2013; 34:42.

[30] Gowani ZS, Sathiyakumar V, Holt GE. Osseous Sarcoidosis. JBJS Rev. 2015;3(4):1.

Chapter 5

Radiation Patterns of Modern Sarcoidosis (Alphabet)

Aleksandra Speranskaia

Abstract

Radiation diagnostics of sarcoidosis in modern conditions is CT, supplemented by radionuclide studies (SPECT, PET), ultrasound, MRI. The paper describes the classic signs of pulmonary sarcoidosis (according to the Statement on Sarcoidosis, 1999), which have changed their characteristics due to the widespread use of CT: variants of lymphadenopathy, dissemination, interstitial involvement. New unfavorable forms of thoracic sarcoidosis are discussed: fibrous sarcoidosis (with a description of the variants of sarcoid fibrosis and their differences from other progressive pulmonary fibrosis) and progressive sarcoidosis (possible causes and patterns). Radiation semiotics of extrapulmonary and comorbid manifestations is touched upon.

Keywords: pulmonary sarcoidosis, systemic sarcoidosis, comorbidity in sarcoidosis, radiation diagnostics, computed tomography

1. Introduction

Sarcoidosis is a polysystemic inflammatory disease of unknown etiology, related by its morphological characteristics to the group of lymphotropic granulomatosis with the formation of noncaseating granuloma, most often the disease reveals, itself as pulmonary sarcoisosis (PS) manifestations [1, 2]. The clinical and radiation symptoms of PS are well studied and defined by the American Thoracic Society (ATS), the World Association for Sarcoidosis and Other Granulomatous Diseases (WASOG), the European Respiratory Society (ERS) and the Russian Respiratory Society [2–4]. On the basis of the traditional X-ray picture of the process, Scaddıng J.G. [5], identified 5 stages of PS, which are used to this day, in a modified version of the assessment by computed tomography (CT). In recent decades, due to the widespread use of CT in patients with PS, there have been revealed changes in the lungs that are not characteristic of this disease and go beyond the stages of its generally accepted radiological classification. According to various authors, the frequency of atypical forms of PS varies from 2–25% or more of all detected cases [6, 7]. In recent decades, there has been an increase in the number of cases of atypical and progressive variants of the course of sarcoidosis, including the formation of fibrosing sarcoidosis of the lungs, damage to vital organs (kidneys, heart, central nervous system) requiring transplantation, and an increase in mortality from sarcoidosis [8, 9]. The ineffectiveness of the treatment has led to the identification of a separate form - refractory sarcoidosis [10]. Most often, sarcoidosis is treated by pulmonologists (since the main manifestation of the disease is PS), a thoracic radiologist who is well aware of the radiation semiotics of disseminated lung processes works with them. However, sarcoidosis is systematic, which requires a pulmonologist to know about possible variants of damage to other organs and systems, and from a radiologist about the radial signs of their damage, the ability to analyze multimodal studies and draw up an optimal radiation algorithm to identify all systemic changes [11]. The incidence of organ damage in sarcoidosis varies across studies, which makes these figures not very reliable (this is probably due to the use of hospital design in most studies, which includes patients with sarcoidosis observed in certain clinics; studies using population design, based on national or regional registers are considered to be the best). It is clear that the likelihood of extrathoracic lesions is very high and underestimated, since they are mostly favorable, asymptomatic (like most of the PS). Isolated extrathoracic lesions in sarcoidosis are very difficult. They mimic various diseases, are poorly recognized without the support of a pulmonologist, are confirmed only morphologically, are often the reason for multiple revisions of morphological data (they will not be considered in this study). The multisystem nature of the lesion can lead to a significant decrease in the patient's quality of life [3]. Extrathoracic lesions in sarcoidosis require additional examination under the supervision of a physician of the relevant specialty. Now, the criteria for cardiosarcoidosis and neurosacoidosis have been published; there are no clear recommendations on the volume and methods of radiation studies in other localizations. Thus, in general clinical practice in the absence of symptoms, a basic eye examination is proposed for screening ocular sarcoidosis, a basic serum creatinine test for screening renal sarcoidosis, a serum alkaline phosphatase test for screening liver sarcoidosis, an ECG for detecting possible heart damage [4]. In determining the typical radiation semiotics of damage to various organs in sarcoidosis, the structured Delphi methodology is used, when the agreement of more than 70% of experts allows a consensus to be reached. This is necessary because a radiologist should be a member of a multidisciplinary team dealing with a patient with sarcoidosis, know the clinical manifestations, possible variants of systemic damage and the optimal radiation algorithm for examining patients with different risks.

While proceeding clinically favorably, sarcoidosis does not really bother the patient, however, comorbid lesions (neoplasms, infectious processes, PE) change both the clinical picture of the disease and its radiation signs [12, 13]. The different types of dissemination seen on CT scan suggest a comorbidity is present. To simplify the assessment of systemic damage in sarcoidosis, attempts have been made to create diagrams that simplify the diagnosis. So, in the work of Schupp J.C., et al. [14], five clinical clusters of sarcoidosis were proposed: (1) damage to the abdominal organs, (2) damage to the eyes, heart, skin and central nervous system, (3) damage to the skeletal muscle and skin tissue, (4) involvement of the pulmonary and intrathoracic lymph nodes, and (5) extrapulmonary involvement. In 2014, the World Association for Sarcoidosis and Other Granulomatous Diseases (WASOG), according to the Delphi study, proposed a probability scale [15]: certain: the likelihood of sarcoidosis causing this manifestation is at least 90% (e.g.: uveitis, bilateral hilar lymphadenopathy, perilymphatic foci on chest CT); probable: the probability of sarcoidosis is 50–90% (for example: paralysis of the seventh cranial nerve, edema of the lacrimal gland, localization of the process in the upper lobes or diffuse peribronchovascular infiltrates); possible: the probability of sarcoidosis is less than 50% (for example: arthralgias, localized infiltration on radiographs). However, in practice, the use of these criteria is not always convenient. Studies in systemic and comorbid sarcoidosis suggest radiation multimodality (MRI, PET, SPECT, 67 Ga scintigraphy), however, CT with its various techniques (HRCT, functional tests, CT angiography) remains the main and at the same time expert method for its diagnosis, which allows and qualitatively answer the questions of the pulmonologist. The article discusses the changes detected during routine CT examination of patients with sarcoidosis, to which a radiologist should draw the attention of the pulmonologist. These findings can change the tactics of patient management and require additional radiation studies.

2. Radiation patterns of modern sarcoidosis (alphabet)

We analyzed the data of radiological studies of 873 patients observed with a diagnosis of sarcoidosis from 2006 to 2021 at the St. acad. I.P. Pavlova. The observation period ranged from 6 months to 22 years. The average age of the patients was 47.2 ± 10.2 years (f / m - 500/373). All patients underwent CT, a pulmonary function tests (PFTs), and echocardiography, in some patients, if necessary, additional radiation studies (MRI, PET, SPECT) were performed. CT data revealed a number of radiation signs of typical (determined by WASOG) and not contradicting (probable and possible by WASOG) PS, which a radiologist needs to know to interpret radiation data correctly. The typical nature of the lesion suggests the possibility of making a diagnosis without biopsy (since even the most benign biopsy options are not desirable due to the development of scars at the site of the surgical injury and the likelihood of a decrease in FVC and DLCO). Radiation signs that do not contradict the manifestations of sarcoidosis require the convening of a multidisciplinary council and a decision to conduct histological verification, atypical radiation manifestations need to be supplemented with morphology. An analysis of the results of radiation research revealed the following radiation features of modern PS:

The defeat of the intrathoracic lymph nodes: typical (58.6%) were symmetrical lesions of the peritracheobronchial, paraaortic, intrapulmonary groups (with the obligatory involvement of bronchopulmonary lymph nodes), the absence of necrotic changes in the structure, the preservation of the integrity of the lymph node capsule, the preservation of the surrounding cellular spaces (**Figure 1a**), the absence of compression adjacent vessels and bronchi even with a large increase in lymph nodes (**Figure 1c**), uniform accumulation of contrast agent in them during all phases of intravenous bolus contrast enhancement (**Figure 1a**) and high metabolism of 18FDG on PET (**Figure 1b**). Not contradicting the diagnosis of sarcoidosis is the presence of calcifications in the structure of the lymph nodes (25.2%) (**Figure 1d**), the asymmetry of their lesions (5.0%) (**Figure 1e**), the lesion of non-characteristic groups (retrosternal, paraesophageal) in combined with the defeat of typical groups (2.3%) (**Figure 1f**).

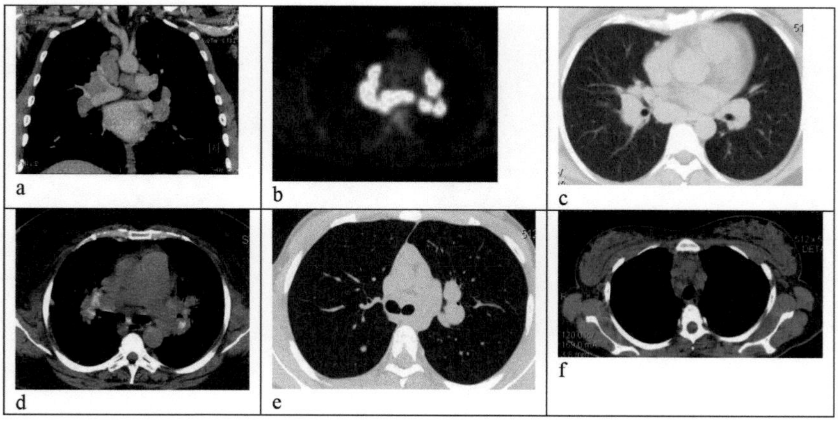

Figure 1.
Radiation picture of the defeat of the lymph nodes with PS (explanations in the text).

Lung lesion with PS consists of two components: the presence of foci and lesions of the interstitium. **Perilymphatic foci were typical** - small (up to 3 mm), of the same type, along the interlobular septa, along the bronchi, vessels, pleura (46.3%) (**Figure 2a**), large foci of irregular oval or trapezoidal perilymphatic arrangement (67.0%) (intrapulmonary lymph nodes), which regressed more slowly than other foci (Figue 2b), fusion of small foci into large ones with indistinct contours (17.1%) (symptom of "galaxy") (**Figure 2c**), fusion of foci into peribroncho-vascular masses - sarcoids (11.9%) (**Figure 2d**). Not contradicting the diagnosis of sarcoidosis is the identification of flat subpleural foci (2.2%) (plaques) (**Figure 2e**), and the presence of calcifications in the foci (1.2%) (**Figure 2f**). The presence of cavities in the foci (0.2%) also did not contradict the diagnosis of sarcoidosis: Patient A., 23 g. 2008 (**Figure 2g**) - typical intrathoracic lymphadenopathy,

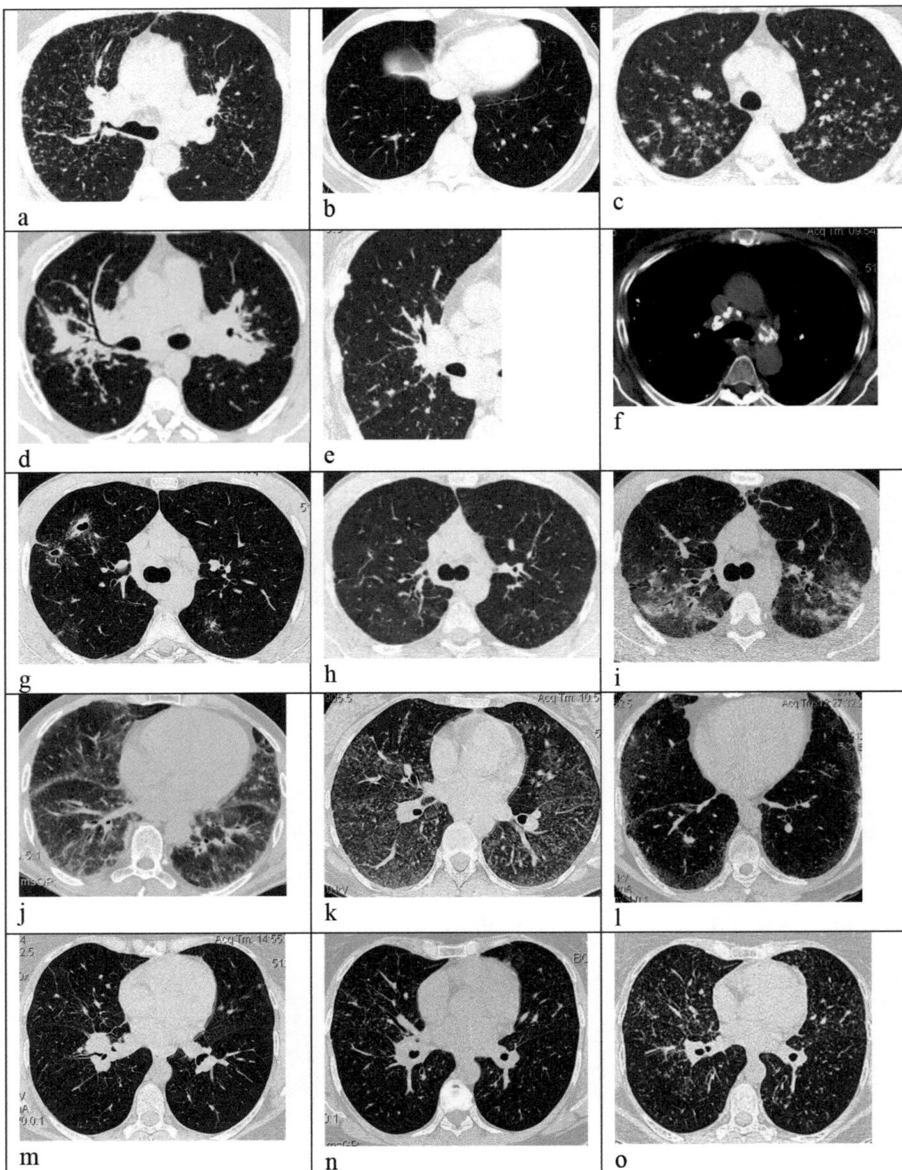

Figure 2.
Radiation picture of lung lesions with PS (explanations in the text).

perilymphatic dissemination with the formation of a symptom of "galaxy", cavities in the foci, 2011 (**Figure 2h**) - regression after steroid therapy with preservation of post-sarcoid perilymphatic fibrous foci, 2013 (**Figure 2i**) progression of the process: an increase in perilymphatic dissemination, edema of the peripheral pulmonary interstitium, the formation of sarcoids. **The lesion of the interstitium** in sarcoidosis can be both of temporary (edema, cell infiltration) and of permanent character (fibrosis) character. Sarcoidosis is characterized by a lesion of the central interstitium with the presence of peribronchovascular "couplings" and sarcoids, damage of the peripheral interstitium (thickening of the interlobular - the wall of the secondary pulmonary lobe and intralobular - acinar septa) is not typical and is an unfavorable symptom that predicts a high likelihood of developing respiratory insufficiency at advanced stages. **Manifestations of sarcoid alveolitis** (10.2%) - compaction of the peripheral pulmonary interstitium of the "ground glass" type, due to the presence of edema and cellular infiltration before the formation of granulomas (**Figure 2j**), or the presence of small perilymphatic foci in the wall of the alveoli (**Figure 2k**) with the possibility of forming fibrosis of the peripheral interstitium (**Figure 2l**). Persistence and increase in edema of the peripheral pulmonary interstitium in sarcoidosis is an unfavorable scenario for the development of the disease, leading to the formation of interstitial fibrosis: Patient K., 49 years old. 2016 (**Figure 2m**), 2018 (**Figure 2n**), 2020 (**Figure 2o**), the progression of the process: regression of lymphadenopathy, an increase in perilymphatic dissemination, edema of the peripheral pulmonary interstitium with the formation of fibrosis, in 2020. - the appearance of shortness of breath, dry cough, a decrease in DLCO to 68% of D. Not contradicting the diagnosis of sarcoidosis is the asymmetry of the lesions of the lung tissue and interstitium (7.2%) (**Figure 2a**).

The transition of PS in stages III and IV is accompanied by fibrosis processes (which, in a number of patients, requires the inclusion of the disease in the category of progressive pulmonary fibrosis). Typical are **fibrotic changes** in the central pulmonary interstitium (at the sites of granuloma localization) with the formation of peribronchovascular fibrous couplings (4.7%) (they differ little from sarcoids, which can regress; within 6 months) with the formation in these areas of traction bronchiectasis of large bronchi (since these are the basal regions), a decrease in the volume of the upper and middle pulmonary fields, in contrast to IPF, in which the lower lobes are more affected. The type of pulmonary volume reformatting is better seen when constructing image reformation (MPR, MinP). Calandriello L., Walsh S.L.F. [16] suggest that posterior displacement of the main or upper lobe bronchus with a decrease in the volume of the posterior segments of the upper lobes is a typical feature of fibrous sarcoidosis. The volume of fibrosis of the lung tissue in stage IV PS is very different: minimal "gentle" fibrous changes of a linear nature (**Figure 3a**), peribronchovascular fibrous couplings (**Figure 3b**), massive peribronchovascular fibrous changes, forcing to change the course of the vessels in the anterior regions to rounded ("vortex" symptom) (**Figure 3c**).

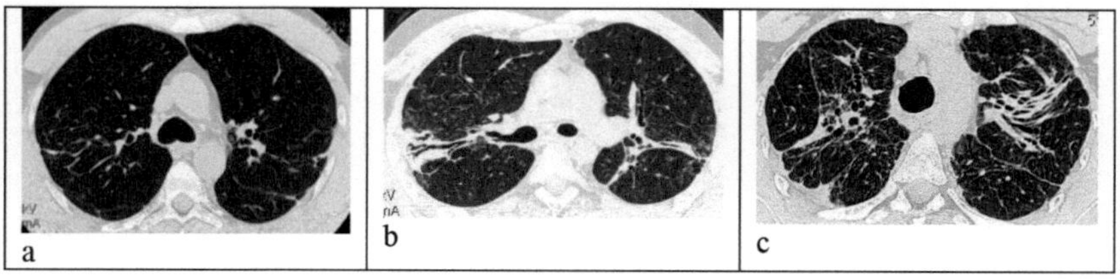

Figure 3.
Radiation picture typical fibrotic changes in PS (explanations in the text).

Not contradicting the diagnosis of sarcoidosis is the identification of a "honeycombing lung", which is rarely observed (1.9%), has a short length and can be localized both in the subpleural and in the basal regions. Preservation of lymphadenopathy and perilymphatic foci is possible at III and IV stages of the disease These forms belong to the unfavorable variants of the clinical course - fibrosing and progressive sarcoidosis. According to Xu L. et al. [17], in contrast to the "honeycombing" in the case of usual interstitial pneumonia (UIP), the "honeycomb" in PS is located centrally and is accompanied by traction expansion of large bronchi (bronchiectasis). It was noted that fibrous and active granulomatous patterns are present in the final stage of PS. Abehsera M. et al. [18] believe that two main models of fibrosing sarcoidosis of the lungs have characteristic radial and functional features: in peribronchovascular fibrosis, obstructive disorders in PFTs with a decrease in FEV1, an increase in OOL, with the formation of a "honeycombing lung" - restrictive disorders with PFTs with a decrease in FVC, DLCO. They also noted that progressive pulmonary sarcoidosis was characterized by the presence of chronic Aspergillus or bacterial infection. D. Valeyrea et al. [19] highlighted the same two main CT patterns of progressive pulmonary sarcoidosis with different functional profiles, noting that they may be with or without signs of activity, concluding that an algorithm based on pulmonary function and CT, allows predicting survival in progressive sarcoidosis. According to our data, 8.9% of patients had a severe course of the disease with dyspnea and radiation signs of fibrosis, which were not typical for the classical version of the course, the traditional radiation pattern and the existing X-ray classification of PS. Our analysis allowed us to identify several models of atypical pulmonary sarcoidosis.

Model of interstitial edema (IE): edema and cellular infiltration of the peripheral pulmonary interstitium (1.5%) was manifested by the presence of small perilymphatic dissemination, merging into a picture similar to the manifestations of interstitial pulmonary edema (clinically also similar to it - shortness of breath, dry cough). Perhaps the fibrous form of sarcoidosis is the outcome of the interstitial-edematous form in patients who did not receive adequate timely therapy, or the result of a comorbid course of sarcoidosis (with viral pneumonia, concomitant occupational pathology) (**Figure 4a**).

Model of idiopathic pulmonary fibrosis (IPF) - fibrosis of the peripheral pulmonary interstitium (1.0%): persistent CT-picture of "ground glass" opacity

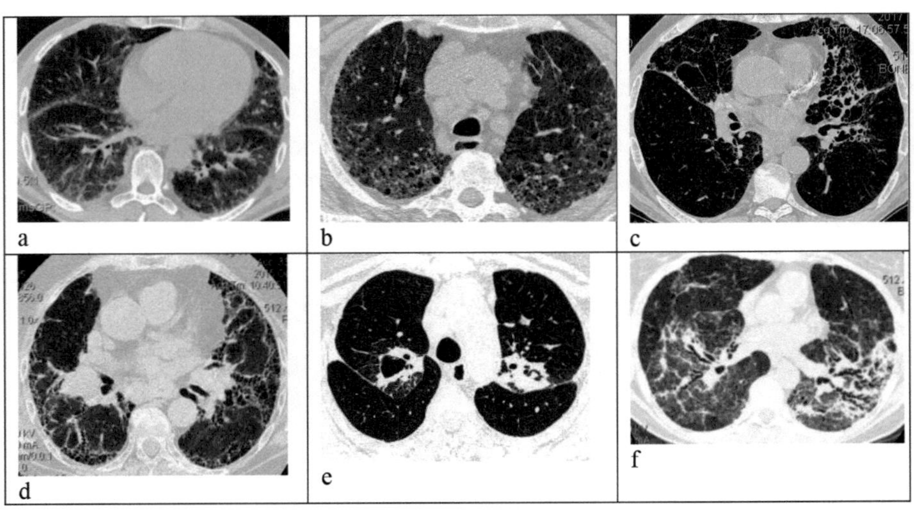

Figure 4.
Radiation picture of possible fibrotic changes in PS (explanations in the text).

(intralobular fibrosis), traction bronchiolyectasis, "honeycombing lung" in combination with lymphadenopathy of the peritracheobronchial groups. With the IPF model of sarcoidosis, there were noticed less severe than with IPF clinical symptoms (moderate dyspnea), a positive reaction to steroid therapy (probably as a result of regression of sarcoid granulomas that exist even at advanced stages of the process), moderate restrictive disorders in PFTs: decrease in DLCO to 55% of D, CT-signs of pulmonary hypertension (SDPA 30.3 + 3.8 mm Hg). Morphological examination revealed manifestations of fibrosing lung disease (fibrosis of the alveolar septa, formation of a "honeycomb lung") and sarcoid granulomas (**Figure 4b**).

Model of hypersensitive pneumonitis (HP) - fibrosis of the central interstitium (1.3%). In the areas of peribronchovascular fibrosis typical for PS, the presence of a "honeycomb lung" with "honeycombs" of a large size was noted. These patients were also characterized by a long-term slow decrease in DLCO (up to 65% of D) and the associated gradual deterioration of health with an increase in shortness of breath and dry cough (**Figure 4c**).

PP + IPF model - fibrosis of the central and peripheral interstitium (0.9%). Fibrosis and "honeycomb" in the upper-posterior basal regions were combined with the presence of "honeycomb lung" in the subpleural areas. Changes of this type were accompanied by pronounced clinical changes (shortness of breath, decreased exercise tolerance, dry cough), the formation of severe pulmonary hypertension (with an increase in systolic pressure in the pulmonary artery to 62 ± 17 mm Hg), a decrease in DLCO (up to 50% of D) (**Figure 4d**).

The model of pneumoconiosis is a fibrocavitary form of PS (1.1%). The formation of cavities in the "sarcoids" (as a result of trophic disorders, or secondary sarcoid vasculitis). The shape of the cavities is irregular, the wall is varied. In some patients, there was a rapid regression of the process when steroid therapy was prescribed. In some patients, the changes progressed. Clinically, it proceeded calmly in most of the patients, in a number of patients it was accompanied by hemoptysis (**Figure 4e**).

A model of progressive PS (3.0%) - a combination of all stages at the same time - lymphadenopathy of the peritracheobronchial groups typical for sarcoidosis, perilymphatic dissemination in the lung tissue, massive fibrous changes of a severe nature in the upper-posterior basal regions on both sides with the formation of traction bronchiectasis. Clinically, these patients had a chronic recurrent unfavorable course of the disease, with wave-like radial changes in the increase and regression of perilymphatic dissemination and lymphadenopathy, were steroid -dependent - more often they were not treated at all (**Figure 4f**).

According to M.H. Jeon, et al. [12], interstitial lung disease with pulmonary fibrosis and pulmonary hypertension was associated with increased mortality, with pulmonary fibrosis accounting for 9.0% of deaths in sarcoidosis. According to Sève P., et al. [20] fibrotic changes on CT in sarcoidosis correlate with PFTs, 6-minute walk test data (6MWT) and the results of the St. George respiratory questionnaire. Thus, a decrease in the ratio of the forced expiratory volume in one second (FEV1)/FVC may be associated with significant deformation of the bronchi, their stenosis due to fibrosis, due to diffuse bronchial granulomatosis, compression of the bronchi with a significant increase in the lymph nodes of the mediastinum, and as a result granulomatous bronchiolitis or bronchial hyperreactivity. Low DLCO values may result from diffuse parenchymal lesions or sarcoid alveolitis.

Calandriello L., et al. [21] write about new trends in the assessment of SP, pointing to new directions: attempts to assess the state of the lung tissue in sarcoidosis using artificial intelligence (radiomics), the wider use of low-dose CT and MRI programs of the chest.

The algorithm of radiation examination for sarcoidosis suggests performing CT to assess intrathoracic changes with the analysis of signs of damage to the organs of the upper abdomen included in the scan area (liver, spleen, lymph nodes, kidneys), supplemented by ultrasound of the abdomen, if necessary, CT examination of the chest and abdomen in the conditions of intravenous bolus contrast enhancement and the use of MRI, PET, SPECT with gallium as reserve methods for assessing the systematicity of the lesion and comorbidity. The decision to appoint additional radiation studies is made by a multidisciplinary council. According to Kobak S. [22], the prevalence of extrapulmonary sarcoidosis is up to 80%. However, it is not known how to assess the systemic nature of the lesion, because almost all patients have minimal extrathoracic radiation and clinical manifestations. It is believed that the skin, eyes, heart and musculoskeletal system are the most commonly affected organs after the lungs. There were reported rare lesions of the gastrointestinal tract and isolated cases of sarcoidosis of the prostate, bladder, bone marrow and thyroid gland. Multiple organ damage is always chronic and more severe, and can lead to a serious disability or potentially fatal consequences. At the same time, according to Jeon M.H., et al. [12], there is no data on a significant difference in PFTs indicators in patients with and without systemic manifestations. According to C.-W. Li, et al. [23], patients with PS and extrapulmonary lesions had more pronounced changes in CT examination in patients with stage II of PS. It is not known which of the combinations of PS and systemic manifestations are the most dangerous. According to our data, systemic lesion in PS is accompanied by changing the favorable course of the disease to a more severe one, symptoms of damage to other organs come to the fore, but the pulmonological multidisciplinary council continues to play a decisive role in the diagnosis. Thoracic changes are the most specific and make it possible to make a diagnosis, while extrathoracic changes may be similar to other processes. Most of the extrathoracic changes are clinically as favorable as classical PS and are detected by chance during additional studies (ultrasound, CT, MRI of the abdomen and pelvis). Others have a vivid clinical picture (neurosarcoidosis, sarcoid cirrhosis of the liver, sarcoid sialoadenitis, sarcoid uveitis), and some may manifest as sudden death (cardiac sarcoidosis). In all cases, the X-ray archive is very important, since at the time of extrathoracic symptoms, PS as a rule has already been delitescent for some time and can be identified retrospectively, even if it was overlooked in the initial analysis. Numerous attempts have been made to combine the symptoms of damage to different organs in sarcoidosis [9, 11, 14, 22, 23]. According to our data, the most frequent X-ray findings during chest CT were extrathoracic lymphadenopathy and damage to the parenchymal organs of the abdomen.

Extrathoracic lymphadenopathy (7.3%): neck, axillary groups, abdomen, pelvis has always been combined, with intrathoracic changes, according to our data. The characteristics of lymph node lesions were the same as those of intrathoracic ones (multiplicity of affected nodes in the group, no violation of the structure and integrity of the capsule, uniform accumulation of contrast agent in all phases of contrast enhancement, including delayed, high metabolism of 18-FDG on PET). Patient N., 29 years old. Lymphadenopathy of the peritracheobronchial groups, perilymphatic dissemination in the lung tissue are typical manifestations of stage II PS (**Figure 5a**), lesions of the lymph nodes of the extrathoracic groups; axillary (**Figure 5a**), deep and superficial cervical groups on both sides (**Figure 5b**), celiac and retroperitoneal groups (**Figure 5c**).

The lesion of the parenchymal organs of the abdomen in sarcoidosis is a frequent accidental finding during CT of the chest organs, because the liver, spleen and kidneys are partially covered by the scanned area. **Spleen** lesion in sarcoidosis may appear as splenomegaly and localized changes. A study by Tetikkurt C., et al. [24] showed that diffuse spleen lesion was associated with PS and other extrapulmonary

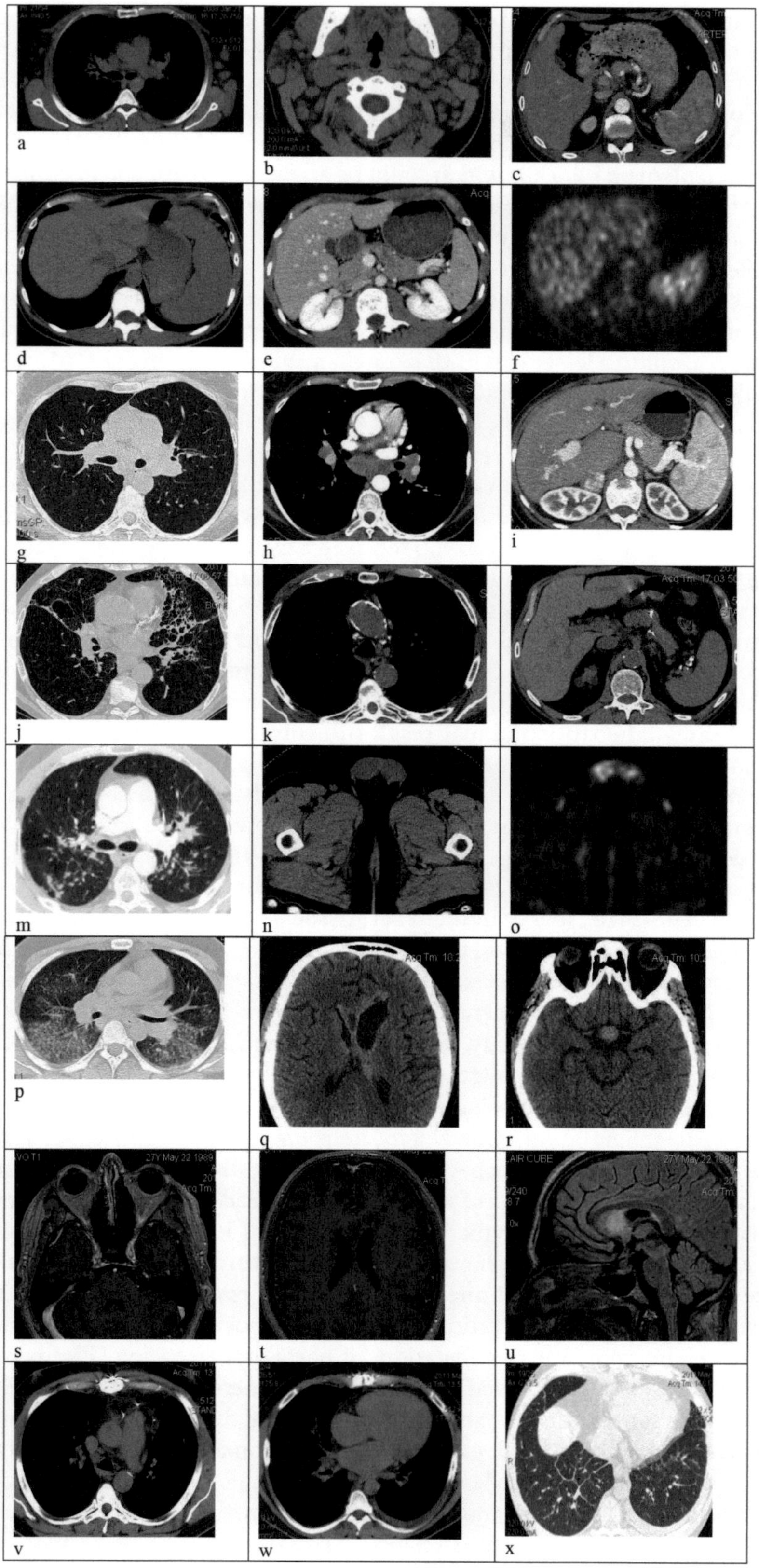

Figure 5.
Radiation picture of systemic manifestations in sarcoidosis (explanations in the text).

manifestations and appears to be a risk factor for chronic sarcoidosis. Changes in the blood count in sarcoidosis (leukopenia, lymphopenia, anemia, thrombocytopenia, and / or pancytopenia) increase the likelihood of bone marrow damage (rare) and the development of splenomegaly. According to our data, damage to the spleen was detected frequently (52.3%). The degree of enlargement of the spleen was different (up to hypersplenism - 2.0%), which could be an indication for splenectomy due to the risk of rupture and the appearance of clinical symptoms - dull ache in the left hypochondrium, shortness of breath, chronic fatigue. Even when the normal size of the spleen was maintained in one third of patients with sarcoidosis, PET showed an increase in the metabolism of 18-FDG, which was a sign of its granulomatous lesion. Rarely foci of low soft tissue density were detected in the spleen, accumulating contrast agent to a lesser extent than unchanged parenchyma (1.6%), regressing independently or during therapy, spleen infarctions (0.3%). The spleen lesion in sarcoidosis - hypersplenism (**Figure 5d**), foci in the spleen (**Figure 5e**), increased 18-FDG in the not enlarged spleen on PET (**Figure 5f**).

The liver is often affected in sarcoidosis. A meta-analysis by E.D. Crouser, et al. [4] showed that liver function tests in sarcoidosis patients were abnormal in 12% of patients, and among those who received a liver biopsy, granulomas were found in 96%. According to Tadros M., et al. [25], in biopsy and autopsy studies of patients with systemic sarcoidosis, liver involvement was found in about 50–80%, some patients may develop end-stage liver disease, and liver transplantation is required. it accounts for about 0.012% of the total number of liver transplants in the United States. P. Sève, et al. [20] note that portal hypertension occurs in 3 to 20% of cases of sarcoid hepatitis and may result from obstruction of the portal venous system due to significant enlargement of the lymph nodes of the hepatic hilum; the development of secondary ischemia, causing cirrhosis and focal fibrosis, or arteriovenous shunts, which increase portal blood flow. In our study, liver damage in sarcoidosis, as well as damage to the spleen, was most often asymptomatic and manifested by hepatomegaly (24.3%), which was accompanied by an increase in the metabolism of 18-FDG, foci of reduced soft tissue density that did not accumulate contrast agent (1.2%). A rare and tragic situation was the development of sarcoid hepatitis and subsequent cirrhosis, identified in 4 patients (0.4%) and manifested by diffuse changes in the liver parenchyma due to small and large-nodular rearrangements, hepatosplenomegaly, portal hypertension, ascites. To assess the progression of these changes, ultrasound elastography and MRI with intravenous contrast enhancement were also used. Patient Sh., 45 years old. Sarcoid cirrhosis of the liver, hepatosplenomegaly, portal hypertension. Lymphadenopathy (significant, symmetrical increase in peritracheobronchial groups, uniform accumulation of contrast agent in them, no signs of compression of adjacent vessels and bronchi), no changes in the lung tissue are typical manifestations of PS I st. (**Figure 5g** and **h**), an increase in the size of the liver and spleen, restructuring of the liver due to the presence of multiple nodes that unevenly accumulate contrast agent, hypertrophy of the caudate lobe are manifestations of sarcoid cirrhosis of the liver; expansion of the portal, splenic veins are manifestations of portal hypertension (**Figure 5i**).

E.D. Crouser, et al. [4] showed that **renal impairment** was detected in 7% of patients with sarcoidosis. Two mechanisms of renal dysfunction in patients with sarcoidosis are considered: parenchymal granulomatous inflammation and changes in calcium metabolism leading to nephrocalcinosis and nephrolithiasis. A meta-analysis by K. Al-Kofahi and P. Korsten [11] showed that 3.6% of sarcoidosis patients had nephrolithiasis at the first visit. They also described rare manifestations of kidney damage in sarcoidosis: pseudotumors or mechanical compression of the urinary tract by significantly enlarged lymph nodes with the formation of hydronephrosis. In our study, such forms of lesion were not identified, the revealed changes were nonspecific: nephrolithiasis (2.8%), secondary renal wrinkling (as a result of a long course of tubolointerstitial sarcoid nephritis) (1.3%). Patient A., 61 years old, histologically verified sarcoidosis, fibrous form of PS IV st., neurosarcoidosis, chronic sarcoid tubulointerstitial nephritis: fibrous manifestations in the lungs that do not contradict PS: "honeycomb" formation in the hilar regions on both sides, minimal hilar lymphadenopathy (**Figure 5j** and **k**), wrinkling of the parenchyma of the left kidney partially included in the scan area (**Figure 5l**).

Polysystemicity presupposes the lesion of other organs, so, according to Lee J.K.T., et al. [26], an autopsy found sarcoidosis of the pancreas, intestines and testicles in 5% of patients. In our study, pancreatic sarcoidosis was suspected in 1 patient with increased metabolism of 18-FDG on PET, intestinal sarcoidosis was not detected, testicular sarcoidosis was an accidental finding during PET in 2 patients (0.2%) (increased metabolism 18 -FDG) and not manifesting clinically. Patient I., 46 years old. Systemic sarcoidosis. Lymphadenopathy of the peritracheobronchial groups, perilymphatic dissemination in the lung tissue are typical manifestations of SP II st. (**Figure 5m**), the absence of anatomical changes in the testes on CT (**Figure 5n**), high metabolism of 18-FDG in them on PET (**Figure 5o**).

Neurosarcoidosis occurs in 3–9% of patients with systemic sarcoidosis (in our study, in 1.1%). Its clinical manifestations are diverse, since any part of the nervous system (brain, meninges, cranial nerves, spinal cord, peripheral nerves) can be affected. CNS lesion predominates over PNS lesion; these lesions usually do not overlap. According to M. Ramos-Casals, et al. [27], systemic manifestations are characterized by a combination of damage to the eyes and the central nervous system, or a combination of damage to the liver and spleen and damage to the peripheral nervous system. According to Acharya N.R., et al. [28], ocular sarcoidosis was detected in 26% of patients with sarcoidosis, with anterior uveitis being the most common pathology (53%). Undoubtedly, the criteria proposed by Stern et al. [29], for a certain, probable and possible neurosarcoidosis will simplify the formulation of this complex diagnosis. Dierkes-Globisch A., et al. [30] showed a statistically significant trend towards a higher incidence of women in patients with CNS lesions and a higher incidence of kidney damage in patients with PNS lesions. Diverse radiation patterns in neurosarcoidosis require a multimodal and multidisciplinary approach. Patient M., 27 years old, complaints about general weakness, unsteadiness when walking, drowsiness, lethargy, rare dry cough, hearing loss in the left ear, thirst up to 5–9 liters per day, polyuria up to 9 liters per day. Lymphadenopathy of the peritracheobronchial groups, perilymphatic dissemination in the lung tissue are typical manifestations of SP II st. (**Figure 5p**). On CT, MRI (**Figure 5q–u**) - periventricular sarcoids (maximally around the anterior horns of the lateral ventricles, more on the left), pituitary sarcoidosis (with manifestations of diabetes insipidus and diabetes), trigeminal nerve on the right.

Cardiac sarcoidosis is an underestimated manifestation of sarcoidosis that can manifest as sudden cardiac death. According to Mehta D. et al. [31], screening for cardiac sarcoidosis includes cardiac MRI (CMR) and PET with 18 F-fluorodeoxyglucose (FDG-PET), ECG, echocardiography. It is noted that patients with delayed accumulation of gadolinium on MRI are at risk of adverse events, even with preserved left ventricular ejection fraction. According to Juneau D. [32], atrial involvement was seen in 9–50% cases of sarcoid. Birnie D.H. [33], notes that coronary arteries are usually normal, but extensive myocardial damage in sarcoidosis can lead to dilated cardiomyopathy. Radionuclide imaging with gallium 67, thallium 201, technetium are alternative tests for diagnosing and monitoring cardiac sarcoidosis that are useful when MRI is contraindicated or unavailable [11]. Patient B., 47 years old, the disease debuted with recurrent pulmonary embolism, repeated infarctions of the anterior wall of the left ventricle with the formation of a left ventricular aneurysm and the development of heart failure refractory to therapy. Six months later, during surgery - linear plasty of the left ventricular aneurysm and removal of the left ventricular thrombus, a biopsy of the left ventricular myocardium was performed, and histological examination revealed epithelioid cell granulomas. After 10 months from the onset of the disease, CT examination of the chest organs revealed borderline mediastinal lymphadenopathy and changes in the lung tissue characteristic of SP II st. (**Figure 5v–x**). Also, there is an expansion of the cavities of the heart, trunk (34 mm) and large branches of the pulmonary artery, manifestations of interstitial stagnation, left-sided pleural effusion - manifestations of cardiomegaly, pulmonary hypertension, heart failure.

The relationship between the radiation signs of **SP and comorbid processes** changes the radiation pattern of both diseases. The most common comorbid processes in sarcoidosis are COPD, neoplasms, infectious processes, IPF and PE. All these comorbid conditions can have manifestations of disseminated chest lesions, complicating the differentiation of these diseases [12, 13]. The most common comorbid pathology in SP is acute PE, recurrent PE (RTE) and pulmonary hypertension, which can be caused by both sarcoidosis itself and chronic embolism (CTEPH). According to E.D. Crouser, et al. [4], echocardiography reveals signs of PH (high systolic pressure in the pulmonary artery) in 29% of patients with sarcoidosis. In his systematic review, Baughman R.P., et al. [34], noted a relationship between PH and the severity of lung disease (a decrease in FVC and DLCO correlated with the degree of PH). This is supported by S. Kobak [22], who noted that in patients with sarcoidosis, DLCO <60% may be a predictor of pulmonary hypertension. At the same time, according to P. Sève, et al. [20], increased pulmonary pressure may be associated with the sarcoid lesion itself: granulomatous lesions of the pulmonary vessels, a consequence of infiltration of the pulmonary parenchyma or compression by enlarged lymph nodes of large branches of the pulmonary artery in the mediastinum.

Acute PE, detected in our study in 3.3% of patients, caused the development of lobular pulmonary infarctions. Such changes can simulate a disseminated process (including sarcoidosis), conceal and be concealed behind sarcoid perilymphatic dissemination: patient K., 57 years old, SP III st., complicated by PE, a marker associated with a decrease in fibrinolytic activity. Multiple contrasting defects of the branches of the pulmonary artery on both sides - thrombotic masses causing their dilation, dilatation of the trunk of the pulmonary artery and its large branches - manifestations of PH (**Figure 6a**), perilymphatic dissemination characteristic of sarcoidosis and lobular infarctions of the lung characteristic of acute PE (**Figure 6b**), the source is a thrombus in the inferior vena cava (**Figure 6c**).

Pulmonary hypertension, often accompanied by IV st., fibrosing and progressive sarcoidosis and was detected in 7.3% of patients: patient D., 59 years old. Grade IV SP, CTEPH. Typical manifestations of SP IV st. are peribronchovascular fibrotic changes with the formation of traction bronchiectasis, volume remodeling with a decrease in the upper lobes and the formation of vascular torsion in the anterior regions - a "vortex" symptom (**Figure 6d**). Parietal contrast defect (long-term thrombotic masses) in a significantly dilated pulmonary artery trunk (**Figure 6e**). High degree of pulmonary hypertension: on a single CT scan, the aortic arch and the extended pulmonary artery trunk (**Figure 6f**).

The combination of sarcoidosis with neoplasms is rare (in our study - in 9 patients (1.0%). Combinations of sarcoidosis with various lymphoproliferative processes (lymphomas, leukemia), neoplasms of various localizations (which apparently are not related to each other), cancers are described. For example, Jamilloux et al. [35] note that lymphoma is a rare cause of death in sarcoidosis. Against the background of perilymphatic dissemination, it is difficult to identify

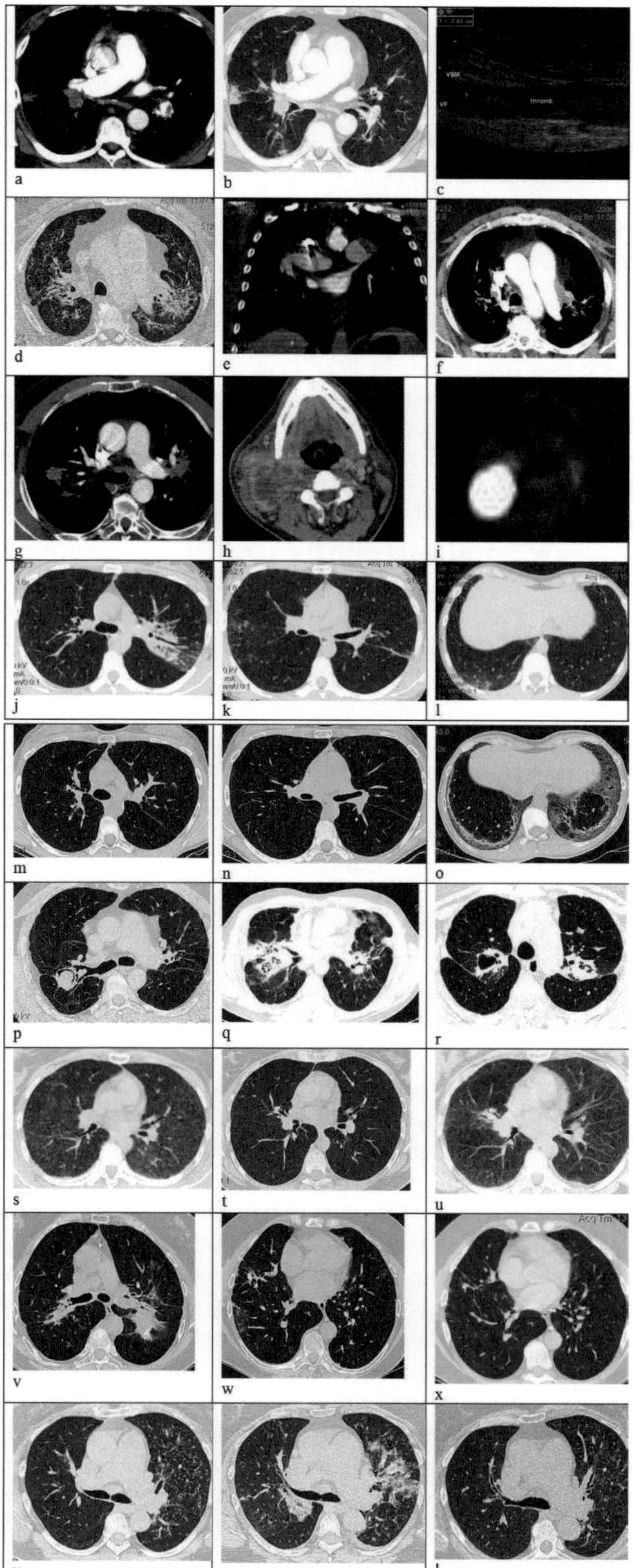

Figure 6.
Radiation picture of comorbid manifestations in SP (explanations in the text).

metastatic lesions, the basis of diagnosis is the hematogenous nature of the spread of metastases (we did not encounter the combination of sarcoidosis with lymphogenous metastatic lesions, perhaps it was not recognized due to the uniformity of the radiation pattern.) In 3 patients (0.3%) with a primary detected neoplasm, signs of sarcoid dissemination were determined, which could be due to the primary detection of sarcoidosis (finding) or a sarcoid reaction with some of the anti-cancer drugs. The use of PET did not help in this situation, because it increased metabolism of 18-FDG in sarcoidosis and oncological processes was equally high: patient I., 45 years old, chest CT - a typical picture of SP II st. - lymphadenopathy of the peritracheobronchial groups, peribronchovascular sarcoids (has had sarcoidosis since 2015, without significant X-ray dynamics) (**Figure 6g**). CT scan of the neck - conglomerate of lymph nodes of the middle deep cervical group on the right: large size, asymmetry, accumulation of contrast agent along the capsule with the presence of irregularly shaped necrotic masses in the center that do not accumulate contrast agent (**Figure 6h**), high metabolism of 18-FDG - poorly differentiated squamous cell cancer of the lateral wall of the oropharynx with secondary lymphadenopathy (**Figure 6i**).

The combination of **sarcoidosis with IPF** (and other progressive pulmonary fibrosis) is a rare, poorly understood situation. It is not clear whether the processes of fibrosis in the lung tissue are triggered by sarcoidosis itself, or whether these are two different diseases. As a rule, carrying out morphological verification also does not clarify the picture, since it identifies both sarcoid granuloma and signs of pulmonary fibrosis. Differential diagnosis with a fibrosing granulomatous process (hypersensitive pneumonitis) is also difficult, because it is often not possible to determine the cause of exogenous exposure. In our study, such a combination was found in 1.9% of patients. Patient V., 34 years old, histologically verified sarcoidosis. On CT from 2017 - perilymphatic dissemination (small foci, sarcoid on the left, manifestations of sarcoid alveolitis in the lower lobe on the right), lymphadenopathy of peritracheobronchial groups (**Figure 6j–l**). On CT from 2019. - multidirectional dynamics - regression of perilymphatic dissemination (traces in the form of small perilymphatic foci of a fibrous nature remain), an increase in interstitial changes in the lower-posterior subpleural regions on both sides - manifestations of progressive pulmonary fibrosis (**Figure 6m–o**).

For sarcoidosis, combinations with pulmonary inflammatory processes, both nonspecific and specific, are rare. The most common were the combination of sarcoidosis with COVID-19 lung damage (5.1%) and the formation of mycetomas in the sarcoid cavities (1.6%). The presence of **mycotic lesions** worsens the course of sarcoidosis due to toxic-allergic effects and the possibility of developing pulmonary hemorrhage. So, Jamilloux et al. [35], note that hemoptysis due to mycetoma can cause death in sarcoidosis. E. Criado, et al. [6], classifies sarcoidosis with manifestations of aspergillosis as an atypical radiation sign of sarcoidosis. The formation of mycetes in the fibrous sarcoid cavities with the appearance of symptoms of "sickle enlightenment" and "rattle" should force a pulmonologist to add antimycotic therapy: variants of mycetes in the sarcoid cavities (**Figure 6p–r**).

There is no increased risk of viral infection in sarcoidosis, however, during the COVID-19 pandemic, some patients with sarcoidosis have suffered this comorbid pathology. An analysis by Robert P. Baughman, et al. of five surveys of US and European survivors of sarcoidosis with COVID-19 [13] provided evidence that the incidence of COVID-19 infection in patients with sarcoidosis was higher than in the general population. They also noted that of the spectrum of immunosuppressive therapies taken by sarcoidosis patients, only rituximab was associated with an increased risk of COVID-19 infection. There was no association between prednisone intake and the development of COVID-19, regardless of the prescribed dose

(≥ 10 and < 10 mg / day). We have identified three main options for the combination of **COVID-19-sarcoidosis**: exacerbation of the course of sarcoidosis against the background of COVID-19 lesions; a combination of radiation signs typical of COVID-19 and sarcoidosis; accidental detection of PS against the background of COVID-19. In patients with sarcoidosis who are prone to developing pulmonary fibrosis, as well as in patients with IPF, COVID-19 could aggravate the course of the process and trigger the course of fibrotic changes.

Patient L., 43, histologically verified sarcoidosis. CT from 2014 (**Figure 6s**) - typical manifestations of PS with the presence of hilar lymphadenopathy and sarcoid alveolitis. CT scan from 2018 (**Figure 6s**) shows regression of the disease. On CT from 06.06.2020 (PCR on RNA SARS-CoV-2 (+) (**Figure 6u**) - bilateral edema of the peripheral and central pulmonary interstitium - CT picture of "ground glass" opacity - manifestations of sarcoid alveolitis overlapping small focal perilymphatic dissemination, lymphadenopathy of peritracheobronchial groups (significant, symmetrical, without violating the integrity of the capsule and the structure of the nodes) - exacerbation of sarcoidosis against the background of COVID-19.

Patient V., 68 years old, histologically verified sarcoidosis. CT scan from 2020 (**Figure 6v**) - typical manifestations of SP III st. with the presence of peribronchovascular fibrotic changes with the formation of traction bronchiectasis, moderate hilar lymphadenopathy, perilymphatic dissemination. Areas of interstitial infiltration in the subpleural regions on both sides - manifestations of COVID-19 lesions (PCR on RNA SARS-CoV-2 (+) (**Figure 6w**). On CT from 2019 (**Figure 6x**) changes characteristic of COVID- 19 were not identified.

Patient A., 62 years old, histologically verified sarcoidosis. CT scan from 2019 (**Figure 6y**) - manifestations of SP II st. with the presence of perilymphatic small focal dissemination, hilar lymphadenopathy, PH. CT from 2020 (**Figure 6z**) - areas of interstitial and alveolar infiltration in the subpleural and nuclear regions on both sides - manifestations of COVID-19 lesion (PCR on SARS-CoV-2 (+) RNA. On CT from 2021 (**Figure 6!**) - regression of COVID-19 lesions, partial regression of perilymphatic dissemination and hilar lymphadenopathy, but an increase in signs of PH, fibrosis of the central and peripheral interstitium.

3. Conclusions

The sarcoid alphabet is an attempt to fully represent the radiation patterns of modern sarcoidosis in images from a to z with an explanation of their features and mechanisms of occurrence. Radiation diagnostics of pulmonary sarcoidosis is now a multimodal study with CT leading (as an expert technique) and supplementing, if necessary, radionuclide studies (SPECT, PET), ultrasound, MRI. Modern classical signs of SP (according to the Statement on Sarcoidosis, 1999) have changed their characteristics due to the widespread use of CT: variants of lymphadenopathy (features of the structure, localization of the affected lymph nodes), perilymphatic dissemination (manifestations of sarcoid alveolitis, types of foci), lesions pulmonary interstitium. Radiation patterns of unfavorable forms of SP were revealed: fibrosing sarcoidosis (with a description of the variants of sarcoid fibrosis and their difference from other progressive pulmonary fibrosis) and progressive sarcoidosis (with the identification of possible causes of its occurrence and radiation patterns). For the convenience of interpreting changes in SP detected by CT, we proposed models of unfavorable forms of SP: interstitial edema (IO), idiopathic pulmonary fibrosis (IPF), hypersensitive pneumonitis (PP), their combination, pneumoconiosis and progressive SP. It was noted that the model of interstitial edema in SP is often combined with multisystem lesions (eyes, kidneys), and has a high risk of developing interstitial fibrosis (transition to the IPF model). The main points to which a radiologist should draw a pulmonologist's attention when performing a CT scan of the chest of a patient with sarcoidosis: describe all unfavorable models of sarcoidosis with the formation of fibrosis, expansion of cardiac cavities (indirect signs of cardiac sarcoidosis, especially in young patients, which requires MRI, or PET of the heart), signs of pulmonary hypertension (the causes of which may be vascular lesions in sarcoidosis and PE, which requires CT angiography, or SPECT), enlargement of the spleen (always within the scan area, may indicate additional hematological problems, both associated with sarcoidosis or not), identification of non-lymphotropic disseminations in sarcoidosis (a sign of comorbidity, requires CT in the whole body mode with multiphase contrast). Patients with sarcoidosis are seen by a pulmonologist and a thoracic radiologist, but the polysystemic nature of the lesion requires these specialists to know the signs of extrapulmonary manifestations of sarcoidosis (both clinical and radiation). If you suspect primary extrathoracic sarcoidosis (neurosarcoidosis, sarcoidosis of the kidneys, skin, eyes) in patients observed by doctors of other specialties, it is necessary to include not only a pulmonologist, but also a radiologist in the multidisciplinary consultation. Detection of radiation signs of comorbidity in sarcoidosis is especially important because it leads to a change in the tactics of patient management. The complexity of the layering of different types of pulmonary dissemination and lymphadenopathy and the multisystem nature of the lesion can be fully determined during a multidisciplinary consultation comprised of a pulmonologist and a radiologist with the involvement of an oncologist, neurologist, infectious disease specialist. The accumulation of experience in clinical and radiation examination of patients with sarcoidosis makes it possible to identify unfavorable clinical and radiological forms: fibrosing, progressive SP, as well as to assess its systemic manifestations and comorbidity, which is important for treatment tactics.

Acknowledgements

Deep gratitude to Baranova O.P. – PhD, Senior Scientific Researcher and Scientific Institute of Interstitial and Orphan Diseases of Federal State Educational Institution of Higher Education "First St.-Petersburg State Medical University n.a. academician I.P. Pavlov of Ministry of Health of Russian Federation (Roszdrav)", Deep gratitude to prof. Ilkovich M.M. chef of Scientific Researcher and Scientific Institute of Interstitial and Orphan Diseases of Federal State Educational Institution of Higher Education "First St.-Petersburg State Medical University n.a. academician I.P. Pavlov of Ministry of Health of Russian Federation (Roszdrav)" and his staff.

Conflict of interest

The authors declare no conflict of interest.

DOI: http://dx.doi.org/10.5772/intechopen.99822

Author details

Aleksandra Speranskaia
Radiology and Radiation Medicine, Department of Federal State Educational Institution of Higher Education "First St.-Petersburg State Medical University n.a. academician I.P. Pavlov of Ministry of Health of Russian Federation (Roszdrav)", Russian Federation

*Address all correspondence to: a.spera@mail.ru

References

[1] Il'kovich M.M. (Ed), Baranova O.P. Pulmonary sarcoidosis. In: Il'kovich M.M. Interstitial lung diseases.: GEOTAR-Media; 2016: 163-234 (in Russ).

[2] Hunninghake G.W., Costabel U., Ando M., et al. ATS/ERS/WASOG statement on sarcoidosis: American Thoracic Society/European Respiratory Society/World Association of Sarcoidosis and other Granulomatous Disorders. Sarcoidosis Vasc Diffuse Lung Dis. 1999;16:149-173.

[3] Saketkoo L. A., Russell A.-M., Jensen K., et al Health-Related Quality of Life (HRQoL) in Sarcoidosis: Diagnosis, Management, and Health Outcomes Diagnostics (Basel). 2021 Jun; 11(6): 1089.

[4] Crouser E. D., Maier L. A., Wilson K. C., et al Diagnosis and Detection of Sarcoidosis. An Official American Thoracic Society Clinical Practice Guideline Am J Respir Crit Care Med. 2020 Apr 15; 201(8): e26–e51.

[5] Scaddıng J.G. Prognosis of intrathoracic sarcoidosis in England. A review of 136 cases after five years' observation. Br Med J. 1961;2:1165-1172.

[6] Criado E., Sanchez M., Ramirez J., et al. Pulmonary sarcoidosis: typical and atypical manifestations at High-Resolution CT with pathologic correlation. RadioGraphics. 2010; 30: 1567-1586.

[7] Shahram Kahkouee et al. Serum ACE Level in Sarcoidosis Patients with Typical and Atypical HRCT Manifestation// Pol. J. Radiol. 2016; 81: 458-461 (in Pol).

[8] Cottin V., Muller-Quernheim J. Imaging of sarcoidosis of the airways and lung parenchyma and correlation with lung function. Eur. Respir J. 2012; 40: 750-765.

[9] Belperio J. A., Shaikh F., Abtin F., Fishbein M. C., Extrapulmonary sarcoidosis with a focus on cardiac, nervous system, and ocular involvement EClinicalMedicine. Published online 2021 Jun 27.

[10] Jammal T. E., Jamilloux Y., Gerfaud-Valentin M., Refractory Sarcoidosis: A Review Ther Clin Risk Manag. 2020; 16: 323-345.

[11] Al-Kofahi K., Korsten P., Ascoli C. Management of extrapulmonary sarcoidosis: challenges and solutions Ther Clin Risk Manag. 2016; 12: 1623-1634.

[12] Jeon M. H., Kang T., Yoo S. H., The incidence, comorbidity and mortality of sarcoidosis in Korea, 2008-2015: a nationwide population-based study Sarcoidosis Vasc Diffuse Lung Dis. 2020; 37(1): 24-26.

[13] Baughman R. P., Lower E. E., Buchanan M., Risk and outcome of COVID-19 infection in sarcoidosis patients: results of a self-reporting questionnaire Sarcoidosis Vasc Diffuse Lung Dis. Published online 2020 Dec 16. doi: 10.36141/svdld.v37i4.10726 PMCID: PMID: 33597796

[14] Schupp J.C., Freitag-Wolf S., Bargagli E., et al. Phenotypes of Organ Involvement in Sarcoidosis. Eur. Respir. J. 2018;51:1700991.

[15] Judson M.A., Costabel U., Drent M., et al. The WASOG Sarcoidosis Organ Assessment Instrument: An Update of a Previous Clinical Tool. Sarcoidosis Vasc. Diffus. Lung Dis. 2014;31:19-27.

[16] Calandriello L., Walsh S.L.F. Imaging for Sarcoidosis. Semin. Respir. Crit. Care Med. 2017;38:417-436.

[17] Xu L, Kligerman S, Burke A. End-stage sarcoid lung disease is distinct from usual interstitial pneumonia Am J Surg Pathol 2013; 37(4):593-600.

[18] Abehsera M, Valeyre D, Grenier P, et al. Sarcoidosis with pulmonary fibrosis: CT patterns and correlation with pulmonary function. AJR Am J Roentgenol 2000; 174:1751-1757

[19] Valeyrea D., Nunesa H., Bernaudin J.-F. Advanced pulmonary sarcoidosis Opin Pulm Med 2014, 20:488-495

[20] Sève P., Pacheco Y., Durupt F., Sarcoidosis: A Clinical Overview from Symptoms to Diagnosis Cells. 2021 Apr; 10(4): 766.

[21] Calandriello L., D'Abronzo R., Pasciuto G. Novelties in Imaging of Thoracic Sarcoidosis J Clin Med. 2021 Jun; 10(11): 2222.

[22] Kobak S. Catch the rainbow: Prognostic factor of sarcoidosis Lung India. 2020 Sep-Oct; 37(5): 425-432.

[23] Li C.-W., Tao R.-J., Zou D.-F., Li M.-H. Pulmonary sarcoidosis with and without extrapulmonary involvement: a cross-sectional and observational study in China BMJ Open. 2018; 8(2): e018865.

[24] Tetikkurt C., Yanardag H., Pehlivan M., Bilir M. Clinical Features and Prognostic Significance of Splenic Involvement in Sarcoidosis. Monaldi Arch. Chest Dis. 2017;87. doi: 10.4081/monaldi.2017.893.

[25] Tadros M., Forouhar F., Wu G.Y. Hepatic Sarcoidosis. J. Clin. Transl. Hepatol. 2013;1:87-93.

[26] Lee J.K.T., Warshauer D. M. Imaging Manifestations of Abdominal Sarcoidosis American Journal of Roentgenology January 2004, VOLUME 182NUMBER 1. 2004;182: 15-28.

[27] Ramos-Casals M., Pérez-Alvarez R., Kostov B., Clinical characterization and outcomes of 85 patients with neurosarcoidosis Sci Rep. 2021; 11: 13735.

[28] Acharya N.R., Browne E.N., Rao N., Mochizuki M. International Ocular Sarcoidosis Working Group. Distinguishing features of ocular sarcoidosis in an international cohort of uveitis patients. Ophthalmology. 2018;125:119-126.

[29] Stern B.J., Royal W., Gelfand J.M., et al. Definition and consensus diagnostic criteria for neurosarcoidosis: From the Neurosarcoidosis Consortium Consensus Group. JAMA Neurol. 2018;75(12):1546-1553.

[30] Dierkes-Globisch A., Schneiderhan W., Mohr H.H.. Acute renal failure due to hypercalcemia and peripheral polyneuropathy–rare manifestations of sarcoidosis. Med. Klin. 2000;95(10):583-586.

[31] Mehta D., Lubitz S.A., Frankel Z et al. Cardiac involvement in patients with sarcoidosis: diagnostic and prognostic value of outpatient testing. Chest. 2008;133:1426-1435.

[32] Juneau D., Nery P., Russo J. How common is isolated cardiac sarcoidosis? Extra-cardiac and cardiac findings on clinical examination and whole-body (18)F-fluorodeoxyglucose positron emission tomography. Int J Cardiol. 2018;253:189-193.

[33] Birnie D.H. Cardiac Sarcoidosis. Semin Respir Crit Care Med. 2020;41(5):626-640.

[34] Baughman R.P., Engel P.J., Meyer C.A., et al. Pulmonary hypertension in sarcoidosis. Sarcoidosis Vasc Diffuse Lung Dis. 2006;23:108-116.

[35] Jamilloux Y., Maucort-Boulch D., Kerever S., et al. Sarcoidosis-Related Mortality in France: A Multiple-Cause-of-Death Analysis. Eur. Respir. J. 2016;48:1700-1709.